Trainee Workbook
for
Mental Health Approaches
to Intellectual/Developmental Disability

– SECOND EDITION –

Robert J. Fletcher, DSW, ACSW, LCSW, NADD-CC

Melissa Cheplic, MPH, NADD-CC

Daniel Baker, Ph.D., NADD-CC

Juanita St. Croix, BSc., NADD-CC

Jeanne M. Farr, M.A.

NADD
An association for persons with developmental disabilities and mental health needs.

321 Wall Street
Kingston, N.Y., 12401

Book design by Michael Frazier.

ISBN: 979-8-9853366-3-4
Library of Congress Control Number: 2022931201

Printed in the United States of America

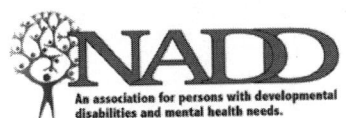

Welcome!

This workbook is a companion to *Mental Health Approaches to Intellectual/Developmental Disability: A Resource for Trainers* and is designed to be given to all participants in workshops using the *Resource for Trainers*.

The material is arranged in 15 modules. It is unlikely that a single training session would attempt to cover every module.

Module I: Understanding Dual Diagnosis Basics
Module II: The Genetics of IDD: Syndromes and Phenotypes
Module III: Comprehensive Assessment Practices
Module IV: Mental Status Exam
Module V: Overview of the Diagnostic Manual for Persons with Intellectual Disability (DM-ID-2)
Module VI: Signs and Symptoms of Mental Illness
Module VII: Positive Support Strategies and Wellness
Module VIII: Crisis Prevention and Intervention: Reducing Risk
Module IX: Adapting Therapy Practices
Module X: Trauma-Informed Supports
Module XI: Childhood and Adolescence
Module XII: Wellness and Aging
Module XIII: Justice System Considerations
Module XIV: The Importance of Direct Support Professionals
Module XV: Collaborating Across Systems

The *Trainee Workbook* contains copies of all the slides that will be used in training but does not include text explaining the slides. That information will be provided by the trainer. The *Trainee Workbook* includes space for you to record your own notes about the material. Each training module includes a pre-test to be taken prior to training and a post-test to be taken after the training.

The *Trainee Workbook* also includes supplemental information for further reflection, study and professional development.

For more resources to empower you in your work with individuals with intellectual or developmental disabilities (IDD) and mental health concerns, please visit **thenadd.org**.

TABLE OF CONTENTS

Introduction:
Cultivating Training Mastery

Introduction:
Cultivating Training Mastery Checklist

General Learning Practices

☐ Cultivate self-awareness. Develop an understanding of your culture (the shared, learned, symbolic system of values, beliefs and attitudes that shape and influence perception and behavior) and how these factors influence your worldview.

☐ Cultivate emotional intelligence. This is defined by Lee Gardenswartz, Jorge Cherbosque and Anita Rowe from the Emotional Intelligence and Diversity Institute (https://www.eidi-results.org/): "Emotional Intelligence is the ability to feel, understand, manage, articulate, and effectively apply the power of emotions as a source of human energy."

☐ Be a continuous learner and keep up to date with the current research on adult learning and the current best practices in the field of study you are training.

☐ Have a system in place (like this checklist) to ensure that the only uncertainty going into the training is what the audience or environment may produce.

☐ Develop your knowledge and experience relating to the material you are training. Be prepared to talk in depth and with familiarity about the content you are teaching.

Preparation Before the Training

☐ Understand the needs, characteristics and makeup of the audience.

☐ Understand the training goals of the organization or individual hiring you to train.

☐ Incorporate effective, emotionally compelling stories and relevant examples throughout your session.

☐ Create a clear outline or agenda for each day that spells out the breaks, lunch and ending times.

☐ Plan to start and end each day with an exercise that brings people together.

☐ Link learning objectives to the organization's (or individual's) identified training needs and goals.

☐ Ensure every topical area leads to the next. (It must all be connected and coherent.)

☐ Incorporate *as many interactive exercises as you can manage effectively*, grouping people differently with each exercise and being cognizant of the hierarchical relationships in the room. Make sure the exercises are concretely linked to the learning objectives.

☐ Ensure training methods attract the engagement of all types of learners and are inclusive of different learning styles.

☐ Make sure the examples, images and vignettes are relevant and that your language is culturally appropriate for each unique group.

☐ Have the chairs and tables organized for maximum group work.

☐ Ensure the lighting is as soft and inviting as the space will allow.

☐ Try to manage the room temperature effectively.

☐ Have good treats and beverages available throughout the session.

☐ Incorporate frequent breaks into the schedule.

☐ Provide a gift or tool to the group (if possible), such as a notebook to record observations or some other item that will remind the participants of the training in the future.

☐ If you have handouts, ensure they are attractive and professional.

☐ Develop a backup plan for presenting your training should technology not work correctly.

☐ If you are not bringing these materials yourself, make sure you have arranged for all the audio-visual equipment (computer, projector, adapter, flash drive with your presentation, microphone, etc.), meeting supplies (flip chart, Post-its, pens, Sharpies, ice-breaker materials, etc.) and training materials (handouts, workbooks, etc.) to be waiting for you when you arrive.

☐ Once the training is designed and planned, create a script or outline for yourself.

☐ Involve people in the process of learning and sharing so the collective experience of the group enhances the learning for everyone involved.

☐ Keep people moving around and interacting as much as you can.

☐ Prepare your evaluation tool for end-of-day feedback from participants. If you are training on behalf of NADD, there will be an evaluation tool to administer. If not, you can create your own or use the evaluation tool included in the appendix of this book.

During the Training

☐ Arrive at the training location very early. This will give you time to make sure everything is working and the environment is as exactly as you had planned (AV and safe electrical cord placement, lighting, temperature, training materials placed where you want them, general room setup, etc.).

☐ To set the tone and create an informal and welcoming environment, greet and spend time with participants as they arrive. Ask them about themselves and what excites them about their work. Modeling this as people enter the room provides a natural segue for you to ask people to share their own experience throughout the day.

☐ Practice active listening and respecting the perspectives of others.

☐ When you first address the group, tell them about yourself, ideally including a relevant short story and elements of your background that relate to the material you are training.

☐ Co-create a set of ground rules to make expectations clear regarding things like being on time, respecting other opinions, texting, taking phone calls or doing other work while in the training.

☐ Model the established ground rules.

☐ Utilize body language consciously (gesture with hands and arms, move around the space effectively, visually connect with all participants, etc.).

☐ Personally connect in some way with each person in the room, so everyone feels seen, heard and valued.

☐ Always scan the room for engagement. Ask for feedback if you sense things are not working well. Change your approach if how you are teaching a segment is not being received as you had hoped.

☐ Let the group know ahead of time that you will seek their feedback at the end of each day so you can learn from their experience and improve your capacity as a trainer.

☐ Create a "parking lot" or place where you can capture questions and issues that need to be addressed.

☐ Near the end of the day, circle back to discuss the "parking lot" items.

☐ Before you end the session and invite people to complete their evaluations, thank them for their engagement, for dedicating the time to increase their skills and for the learning you gained by working with them.

☐ Give participants specific information on how they can contact you or NADD for additional resources or learning opportunities.

☐ At the end of the day, seek the participants' feedback and allow enough time for people to complete the evaluation before they leave the room.

After the Training

☐ Collect the evaluations.

☐ Return the room to its original condition. You may want to ask for volunteers to help you.

☐ Take all feedback and consider each comment for the lessons so you may learn from them and incorporate them into your next training. If there are trends, those are worthy of deep consideration and learning. Isolated comments may not be particularly helpful.

☐ If you are doing a multi-day training, start each subsequent day with a very general summary of the trends of the feedback (not individual comments) and how you are addressing the insights.

Digital Training

☐ If possible, conduct the training on a digital platform that allows for video participation and breakout sessions.

☐ Utilize emotionally compelling stories, videos and pictures, which are even more important when training remotely.

☐ To keep participants focused, break the training modules into small increments of about 20 minutes, with engaging activities between the 20-minute increments.

☐ To ensure participant learning, break up the trainings over multiple days, with no more than four full hours in a day, including breaks.

☐ Be trained and proficient with the digital platform you are using. (This is critical.)

☐ Before the day of your training, practice all aspects and phases of your training to make sure they work effectively (group video engagement, breakout sessions, screen share, etc.).

☐ Be sure you present a professional and calming presence. Don't wear bright colors or extreme patterns. Wearing a pastel color with a gentle neutral background is important.

☐ Be aware of your vocal tone and where your eyes are focused. Be a welcoming presence to those watching and listening.

☐ Add to your opening session a tutorial on the details of the digital platform so participants know how to use the chat function, how to raise their hand to speak, why it is important to remain muted unless speaking, etc.

☐ To maintain a professional atmosphere, incorporate into the tutorial a description of digital etiquette, including how to: position their camera, use the microphone, create the best lighting, ensure their environment is free of distractions, etc.

☐ Convert your evaluation process into an automated survey format and allow for completion after each day of training, so you can learn from participant feedback before you next train.

Module I

Understanding Dual
Diagnosis Basics

Pre-Test

Module I: Understanding Dual Diagnosis Basics

_____ B 1. Which of the following is the most accurate description of a dual diagnosis?
(a) Coexistence of two disabilities: intellectual/developmental disability (IDD) and mental illness (MI)
(b) Coexistence of two or more mental health diagnoses
(c) Coexistence of a mental health disorder and complex behavioral support needs
(d) Coexistence of two or more distinct "personalities"

_____ T 2. True or false: In 2013, the DSM-5 updated terminology from "mental retardation" to "intellectual disability" or "intellectual developmental disorder."

_____ 3. True or false: Adaptive functioning refers to a person's capacity to gain personal independence, based on the person's ability to learn and apply conceptual, social and practical skills in their everyday life.

_____ 4. People who have an intellectual/developmental disability often have impairments of general mental abilities that impact adaptive function, which determine how well an individual copes with everyday tasks in the:
(a) Conceptual domain, the social domain and the practical domain
(b) Conceptual domain, the practical domain and the vocational domain
(c) Practical domain, the conceptual domain and the recreational domain
(d) Conceptual domain, the social domain and the virtual domain

_____ 5. Intellectual/developmental disabilities can be categorized as:
(a) Mild, moderate, profound and extreme
(b) Invisible, moderate, severe and profound
(c) Moderate, profound, debilitating and severe
(d) Mild, moderate, severe and profound

_____ 6. For people who have intellectual/developmental disabilities, mental health disorders can be caused by:
(a) Brain abnormalities
(b) Bio-psycho-social influences
(c) Vulnerabilities from environmental factors
(d) All of the above

_____ 7. True or False: It is likely that about 25% of people who have an intellectual/developmental disability will develop a mental health problem at some point in their lives.

_____ 8. Psychological vulnerability factors for developing mental health challenges for people who have intellectual/developmental disabilities do not include:
(a) Rejection/deprivation/abuse
(b) Life events/separations/losses
(c) Poor self-acceptance/low self-esteem
(d) Autism spectrum disorder and other neurodevelopmental challenges

_____ 9. What might assist a person with IDD through some of their learning issues?
(a) Strategies to gain attention: using the person's name frequently
(b) Positive support strategies
(c) Errorless learning strategies (setting the person up for success)
(d) All of the above
(e) (a) and (b) only

_____ 10. True or false: People who have a dual diagnosis experience similar employment rates and make as much money as those who have an intellectual/developmental disability only.

Slide 1

Module I

**Understanding Dual
Diagnosis Basics**

Slide 2

This module covers basic information about the nature of mental health disorders among persons with intellectual or developmental disabilities (IDD). The following content will be covered: definitions of IDD and mental illness (MI), prevalence, indicators, characteristics, vulnerability factors, and similarities and differences between MI and IDD.

Slide 3

Learning Objectives

- Define "dual diagnosis."
- Describe vulnerability risk factors.
- Articulate the similarities and differences between MI and IDD.

Slide 4

- Coexistence of two disabilities: Intellectual/Developmental Disability (IDD) and Mental Illness (MI)
- Both IDD and mental health disorders should be assessed and diagnosed.
- All needed treatments and supports should be available, effective and accessible.

Slide 5

Terminology

The DSM-5 was published in May 2013 with many changes in diagnostic criteria and terminology.

One of these is the change from the term "mental retardation" from DSM-IV to the term "intellectual disability" or "intellectual developmental disorder." This change better reflects terminology changes by medical, educational and service professionals and advocacy groups.

DSM 5, 2013

Slide 6

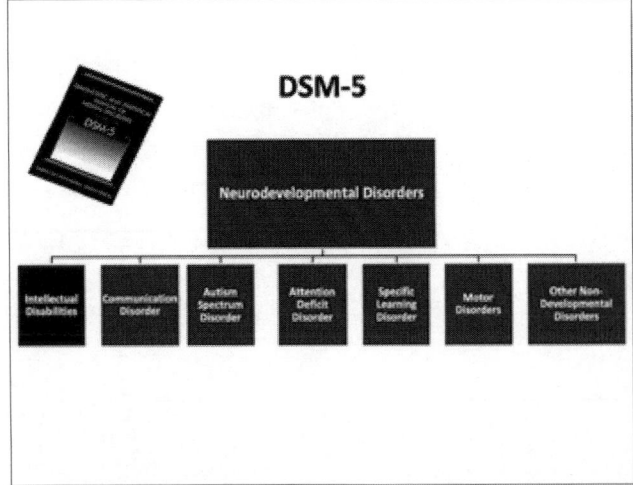

Slide 7

Intellectual/Developmental Disorder

The following three diagnostic criteria must be met:

1. Deficits in intellectual functioning, such as reasoning, problem-solving and planning, abstract thinking, academic learning and learning from experience, confirmed by both clinical assessment and individualized standardized testing.
2. Deficits in adaptive functioning that result in failure to meet developmental and sociocultural standards for personal independence and social responsibility. Without ongoing support, the adaptive deficits limit functioning in one or more activities of daily life, such as communication, social participation and independent living, across multiple environments, such as home, school, work and community.
3. Onset of intellectual and adaptive deficits during the developmental period.

DSM 5, 2013

Slide 8

Disorder Characteristics: Three Domains

Intellectual/Developmental Disorder involves impairments of general mental abilities that impact adaptive functioning in three domains or areas. These domains determine how well an individual copes with everyday tasks:

- **The Conceptual Domain** includes skills in language, reading, writing, math, reasoning, knowledge and memory.

- **The Social Domain** refers to empathy, social judgment, interpersonal communication skills, the ability to make and maintain friendships and similar capacities.

- **The Practical Domain** centers on self-management in areas such as personal care, job responsibilities, money management, recreation and organizing school and work tasks.

DSM 5, 2013

Slide 9

- Self-care
- Language and communication
- Community use
- Independent living skills

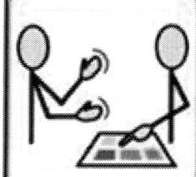

DMHD, 2007

Slide 10

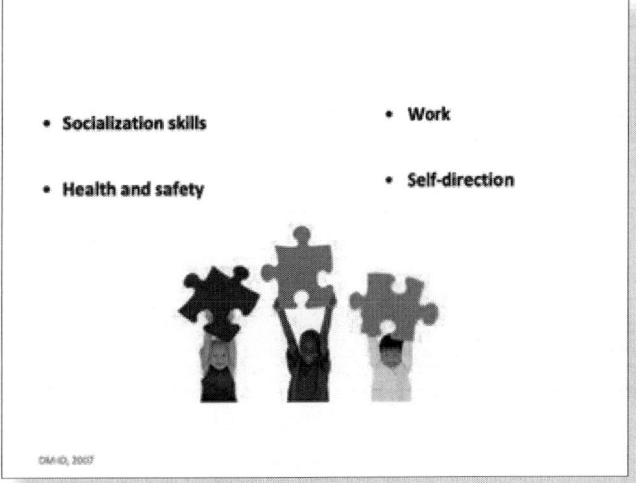

- **Socialization skills**
- **Health and safety**
- **Work**
- **Self-direction**

DM-ID, 2007

Slide 11

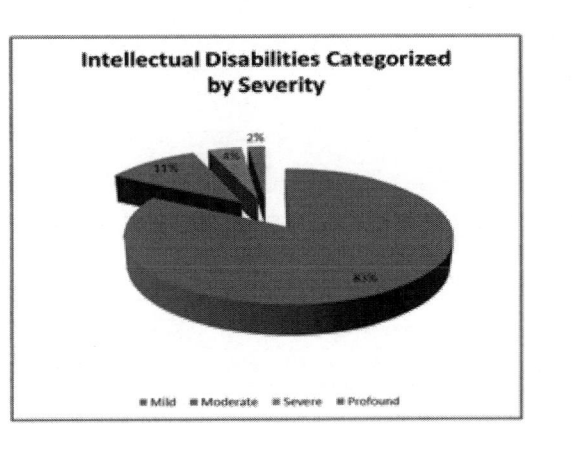

Intellectual Disabilities Categorized by Severity

2%
4%
11%

85%

▪ Mild ▪ Moderate ▪ Severe ▪ Profound

Slide 12

Mild: 80-85 percent of people with IDD:

- Slower-than-normal development in all areas
- Unusual physiology is rare
- Typical skill repertoire includes:
  - Practical skills
  - Literacy skills
  - Tasks of daily living/self-care
  - Social skills

DSM 5, 2013

Slide 13

Moderate: 10-12 percent of people with IDD:

- Noticeable delays, particularly with speech and communication
- May have unusual physiology
- Typical skills repertoire includes:
    - Simple communication skills
    - Simple health and safety skills
    - Some tasks of daily living/self-care
    - Independence in the community in familiar places

DSM 5, 2013

Slide 14

Severe: 3-4 percent of people with IDD:

- Significant delays in some areas
- Delayed motor development
- Limited expressive communication skills
- Typical skills repertoire includes:
    - Daily routines and repetitive activities
    - Less complex tasks of daily living/self-care
    - Social skills with support and supervision

DSM 5, 2013

Slide 15

Profound: 1-2 percent of people with IDD:

- Significant delays in all areas
- Congenital abnormalities present
- Require specialized/attendant care
- May respond to regular physical and social activity
- Need intensive support and supervision to do self-care and activities of daily living

DSM 5, 2013

M
O
D
U
L
E

1

Slide 16

Exercise and Discussion

- What do you know about each of the severity levels of IDD (mild, moderate, severe, profound)?
- What is your personal experience with someone who has a disability?

Slide 17

People occasionally experience mental health problems that may:

- Change the way they think and understand the world around them
- Change the way they relate with others
- Change the emotions and feelings they have

These changes can have a short-term impact on the way they deal with day-to-day life.

However, if the impact is very great (ongoing problems with repeated relapse episodes), then we consider the possibility of mental illness.

Slide 18

- MI is a psychiatric condition that disrupts a person's thinking, feeling, mood or ability to relate to others and can impair daily functioning.
- MI can affect people of any age, race, religion, income or level of intelligence.
- The DSM-5 or the DM-ID provide diagnostic criteria for mental disorders.

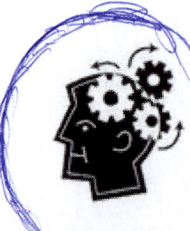

Slide 19

Mental illness is a biological process that affects the brain. Some refer to it as a brain disorder.

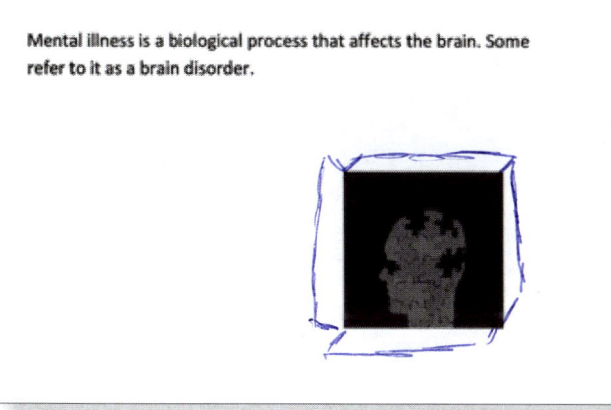

Slide 20

Mental illnesses (mental disorders) can also be defined as a variety of psychiatric conditions that may be a result of vulnerabilities in:

- Environment
- Biology
- Psycho-social factors

DSM 5, 2013

Slide 21

Criteria

1. When behavior is abnormal by virtue of quantitative or qualitative differences.
2. When behavior cannot be explained on the basis of developmental delay alone.
3. When behavior causes significant impairment in functioning.

M
O
D
U
L
E

1

Slide 22

Exercise

What did you learn from this section regarding people who have IDD/MI?

Slide 23

Two to four times a typical population
(Corbett 1979)

32.9% of people with IDD have co-occurring MI
(NCI 2011-2012)

55% of people with IDD have MI
(NCI, 2016)

Slide 24

Total U.S. Population:
(U.S. Census Bureau, Census 2020)
330,017,895

Number of People in Total Population with IDD:
5,280,286
(1.6% – NADD)

Number of People with IDD Who Have MI:
1,737,214
(32.9% of ID – NCI, 2012)

Slide 25

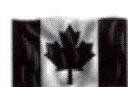

Total Canadian Population
37,766,314
(Government of Canada, Statistics Canada, 2018)

Number of People in the Total Population with IDD:
604,261
(1.6% NADD)

Number of People with IDD Who Have MI:
198,802
(32.9% ID- NCI, 2012)

Slide 26

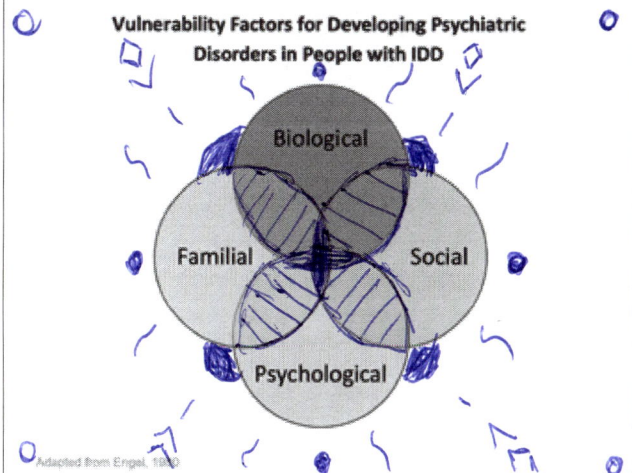

Vulnerability Factors for Developing Psychiatric Disorders in People with IDD

Biological

Familial

Social

Psychological

Adapted from Engel, 1980

Slide 27

People with IDD are at increased risk of developing psychiatric disorders due to complex interaction of multiple factors:

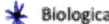 Biological

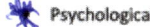 Psychological

Social

Family

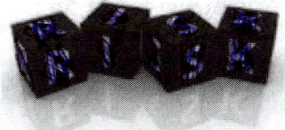

Royal College of Psychiatrists, 2001

Slide 28

Vulnerability factors for psychiatric disorders

Biological

- Brain damage/epilepsy
- Vision/hearing impairments
- Physical illnesses/disabilities
- Genetic/familial conditions
- Drugs/alcohol abuse
- Medication/physical treatments

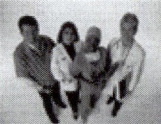

Royal College of Psychiatrists, 2001

Slide 29

Psychological

- Rejection/deprivation/abuse
- Life events/separations/losses
- Poor problem-solving/coping strategies
- Social/emotional/sexual vulnerabilities
- Poor self-acceptance/low self-esteem
- Devaluation/disempowerment

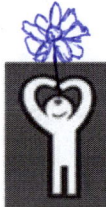

Royal College of Psychiatrists, 2001

Slide 30

Social

- Negative attitudes/expectations
- Stigmatization/prejudice/social exclusion
- Poor supports/relationships/networks
- Inappropriate environments/services
- Financial/legal disadvantages

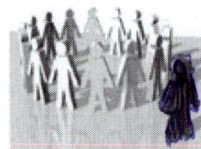

Royal College of Psychiatrists, 2001

MODULE 1

Slide 31

Family

- Diagnostic/bereavement issues
- Life-cycle transitions/crises
- Stress/adaptation to disability
- Limited social/community networks
- Difficulties "letting go"

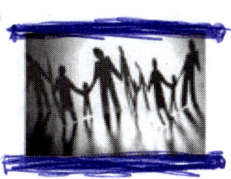

Royal College of Psychiatrists, 2001

Slide 32

Consider This Person

Tran is a 41-year-old woman who was diagnosed with mild IDD at age 12. She has recently moved from her family home to group living after the sudden death of her sister, with whom she spent nearly all her time.

Tran has been refusing to go to bed at night, spending hours awake sitting in the living room of her new home. Normally, Tran is not a fussy eater, but since moving, she has been leaving most of her meal on her plate and declining snacks when offered.

The Direct Support Professionals (DSPs) who support Tran are concerned about her. What do you think Tran could be experiencing?

Slide 33

High Vulnerability to Stress

The impact of a minimally or moderately stressful situation can be experienced as significant.

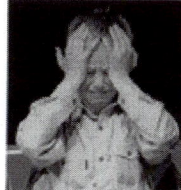

Hartley and MacLean, 2009

MODULE 1

Slide 34

Vulnerabilities in Skill Acquisition

- Challenges with coping skills
- Stress-management difficulties
- Fewer wellness opportunities
- Frequently lack the basic skills required for everyday living, e.g., budgeting money, using public transportation, doing laundry, preparing meals, etc.

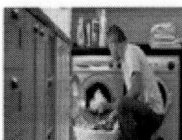

Slide 35

Extreme Dependence

People who have IDD/MI can often experience themselves as quite helpless, thus requiring massive support from families or care providers to live successfully.

Hartley & Maclean, 2009

Slide 36

Difficulty with Interpersonal Relationships

- With some exceptions, people with IDD/MI often have great difficulty in developing and maintaining close relationships with others.
- These interpersonal relationship problems can result in disruption in school, home, work and social environments.

Hartley & McLean, 2009

M
O
D
U
L
E

1

Slide 37

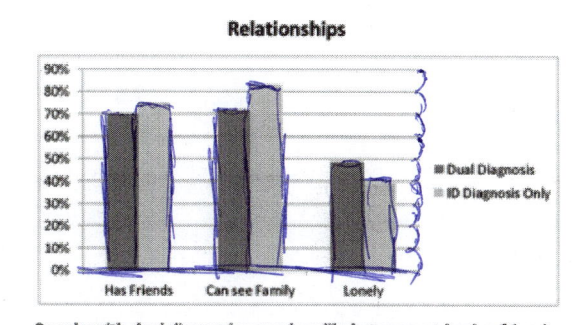

People with dual diagnosis were less likely to report having friends (70% vs. 75%) and being able to see family whenever desired (72% vs. 83%) than were those with IDD only. On the other hand, they were considerably more likely to report feeling lonely (49%) than were people with diagnosis of only IDD (39%).

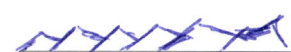

Slide 38

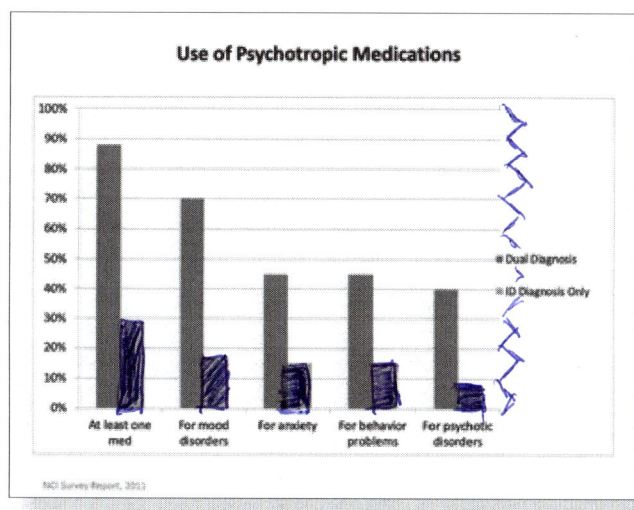

Slide 39

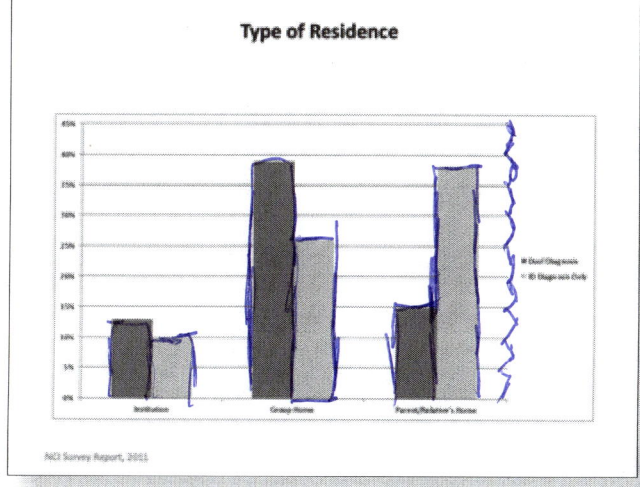

M
O
D
U
L
E

1

Slide 40

Difficulty Working in the Competitive Job Market

People with IDD/MI often have difficulty working in a competitive employment. They may have frequent job changes interspersed with long periods of unemployment.

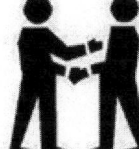

Carter & Wehby, 2008

Slide 41

Employment (community job)

	Hours worked in two weeks	Amount earned in two weeks (USD)	Hourly wage	Earning at or above minimum wage (%)	Length at current job
Dual Diagnosis	30.6	$170	$5.81	35%	56 months
IDD Only	31.5	$201	$6.40	43%	66 months

NCI Survey Report, 2010

Slide 42

- People with IDD/MI may learn more slowly.
- They may have difficulty recalling information—especially newly acquired information.

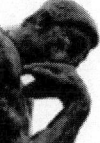

Slide 43

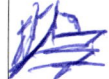
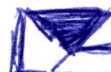

- May have difficulty focusing, may have shortened attention span
- Difficulty in understanding some abstract concepts
- May have difficulty in considering alternative solutions. For example, may see things in black-and-white terms.

Slide 44

- May have difficulty generalizing skills sets
- Developed skill sets may be very task-specific
- May have a passive learning style, which may make it difficult for the trainer to know what information is being retained
- Low expectations due to past difficulties. "Self-fulfilled prophecy" — the individual believes he/she cannot learn, thus preventing learning.

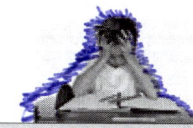

Slide 45

Exercise

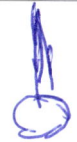
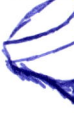

Can you share examples of what might assist a person with IDD through some of the learning issues on the previous slide?

M O D U L E 1

Slide 46

- May repeatedly do or think about the same thing
- Much harder to focus on things that are too difficult
- Problems with cognitive rigidity:
    - Difficulty changing from one task to another
    - Difficulty accepting alternative solutions or explanations
    - Difficulty shifting focus of attention

Slide 47

- Being different from peers
- More experience with losses rather than gains
- Social isolation although mainstreamed
- Rejected by peers
- Failure experiences dominate school histories
- Low social status

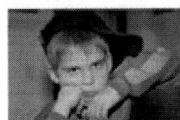

Heiman & Margalit, 1998

Slide 48

- Outer-directed personality orientation — looking to others rather than selves for problem solution
- Very unusual social styles:
    - Too wary or too disinhibited
    - Low expectancy or enjoyment of success

Zigler & Bennett-Gates, 1999

Slide 49

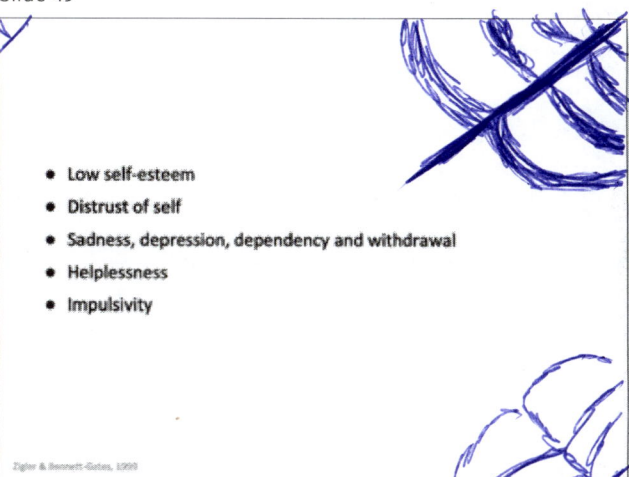

- Low self-esteem
- Distrust of self
- Sadness, depression, dependency and withdrawal
- Helplessness
- Impulsivity

Zigler & Bennett-Gates, 1999

Slide 50

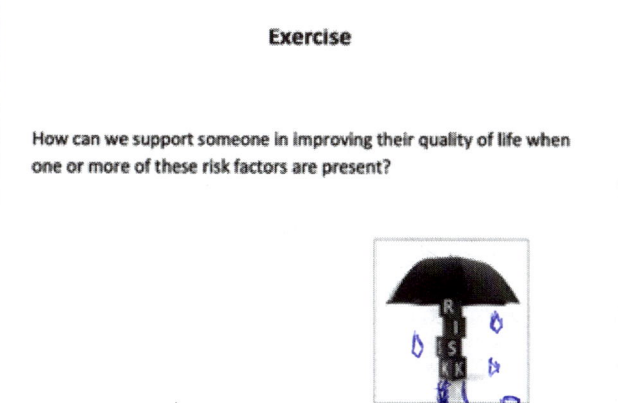

Exercise

How can we support someone in improving their quality of life when one or more of these risk factors are present?

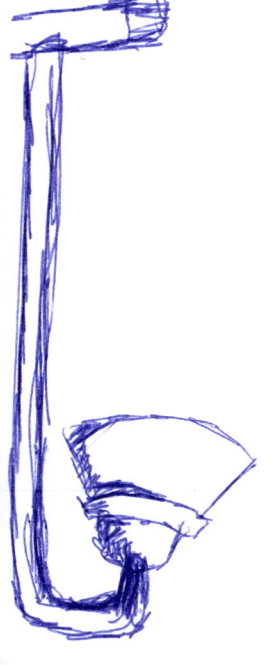

M
O
D
U
L
E

1

Post-Test

Module I: Understanding Dual Diagnosis Basics

_____ 1. Which of the following is the most accurate description of a dual diagnosis?
(a) Coexistence of two disabilities: intellectual/developmental disability (IDD) and mental illness (MI)
(b) Coexistence of two or more mental health diagnoses
(c) Coexistence of a mental health disorder and complex behavioral support needs
(d) Coexistence of two or more distinct "personalities"

_____ 2. True or false: In 2013, the DSM-5 updated terminology from "mental retardation" to "intellectual disability" or "intellectual developmental disorder."

_____ 3. True or false: Adaptive functioning refers to a person's capacity to gain personal independence, based on the person's ability to learn and apply conceptual, social and practical skills in their everyday life.

_____ 4. People who have an intellectual/developmental disability often have impairments of general mental abilities that impact adaptive function, which determine how well an individual copes with everyday tasks in the:
(a) Conceptual domain, the social domain and the practical domain
(b) Conceptual domain, the practical domain and the vocational domain
(c) Practical domain, the conceptual domain and the recreational domain
(d) Conceptual domain, the social domain and the virtual domain

_____ 5. Intellectual/developmental disabilities can be categorized as:
(a) Mild, moderate, profound and extreme
(b) Invisible, moderate, severe and profound
(c) Moderate, profound, debilitating and severe
(d) Mild, moderate, severe and profound

_____ 6. For people who have intellectual/developmental disabilities, mental health disorders can be caused by:
(a) Brain abnormalities
(b) Bio-psycho-social influences
(c) Vulnerabilities from environmental factors
(d) All of the above

M
O
D
U
L
E

1

_____ 7. True or False: It is likely that about 25% of people who have an intellectual/developmental disability will develop a mental health problem at some point in their lives.

_____ 8. Psychological vulnerability factors for developing mental health challenges for people who have intellectual/developmental disabilities do not include:
(a) Rejection/deprivation/abuse
(b) Life events/separations/losses
(c) Poor self-acceptance/low self-esteem
(d) Autism spectrum disorder and other neurodevelopmental challenges

_____ 9. What might assist a person with IDD through some of their learning issues?
(a) Strategies to gain attention: using the person's name frequently
(b) Positive support strategies
(c) Errorless learning strategies (setting the person up for success)
(d) All of the above
(e) (a) and (b) only

_____ 10. True or false: People who have a dual diagnosis experience similar employment rates and make as much money as those who have an intellectual/developmental disability only.

MODULE 1

Supplemental Materials

Module I: Understanding Dual Diagnosis Basics

1. In addition to problems with expressive or receptive language, reasoning problems or difficulty with money management, what else might you observe that indicates a person may have impairments that impact adaptive function?

2. Think about the three criteria for diagnosing mental health problems in a person with IDD:

   - Maladaptive behavior is observed and there is a difference in frequency or content of the behavior from baseline.

   - The maladaptive behavior, which is a change from baseline, is not directly a result of the IDD.

   - Maladaptive behavior, which is a change from baseline, results in impairment in day-to-day functioning over time (Einfeld & Aman, 1995).

   Can you identify someone you currently support or whom you previously supported who may have been experiencing an undiagnosed or misdiagnosed mental illness? On what factors are you basing your conclusion?

3. Several risk factors predispose people with IDD to develop psychiatric disorders. There are biological, psychological and social circumstances that contribute vulnerability to mental health disorders in persons with IDD.

   List a couple of factors for each of these four.

MODULE 1

a. biological factors

_____

_____

b. social factors

_____

_____

c. family factors

_____

_____

d. psychological factors

_____

_____

4. What are the benefits of having a good friend? Of being a good friend?

_____

_____

5. What qualities make someone a good friend to others?

_____

_____

M
O
D
U
L
E

1

6. What skills do you think are needed to develop and maintain good friendships and interpersonal relationships?

    _____

    _____

7   What do you need to do to help someone learn to be a good friend and build strong, positive relationships? Are you able to support people to develop these skills or find a way to develop them?

    _____

    _____

8. What is the value of being employed? What value would employment add to the life of a person with a dual diagnosis?

    _____

    _____

9. There are numerous resources about supported employment for all people with intellectual/ developmental disabilities.

    a. What do you believe are the barriers to meaningful employment for people with IDD?

    _____

    _____

    b. How might you help someone overcome these barriers?

    _____

    _____

Additional Resources

A Summary of Similarities and Differences Between Intellectual/Developmental Disability (IDD) and Mental Illness (MI)

IDD: refers to sub-average functional intellect
MI: has nothing to do with intellect

IDD: incidence: 1 to 2% of the general population
MI: incidence: 16 to 20% of the general population

IDD: present at birth or occurs before age 18
MI: may have its onset at any age

IDD: functional intellectual impairment is permanent
MI: often temporary, may be reversible and is often cyclic

IDD: a person can usually be expected to behave rationally at his or her developmental level
MI: a person may vacillate between normal and irrational behavior, displaying degrees of each

Comparison between IDD and MI

Intellectual/Developmental Disability	Mental Illness
Below-average ability to learn and to use information	Inappropriate thought processes and/or emotions
Before adulthood	Can occur any time in a person's life
Refers to sub-average functional intellect	Has nothing to do with intellect
Lifelong. There is no cure.	May be temporary, cyclic or episodic May be curable
Services involve training and education, not medication	Services involve therapy and medication
Is not psychiatric in nature	Diagnosed illnesses such as depression, schizophrenia, bipolar disorder
Impairments in social skills and adaptations	Does not necessarily impact social competence
Behavior is usually rational	Behavior may vacillate between normal and irrational

M
O
D
U
L
E

1

Signs someone with IDD may have MI

- Increased anxiety, panic or fright

- Excessive reactivity/moodiness

- Hearing, seeing, feeling imaginary things (hearing voices is not the same as talking to oneself for company, to process thoughts or to reduce anxiety)

- Memory problems (worsening memory or change in memory)

- Need for instant fulfillment/gratification

- Accelerated speech patterns

- Unusual sleep patterns (insomnia or lengthy periods of sleep)

- Changes in appetite

- False beliefs (delusional thinking or paranoia)

- Heightened emotional sensitivity

- Decline in personal hygiene

- Self-isolation

- Inappropriate expressive reactions

- Lingering sadness

- Family history of mental illness

- Self-injurious behavior

- A functional or behavioral change

- Suicidal ideation

M
O
D
U
L
E

1

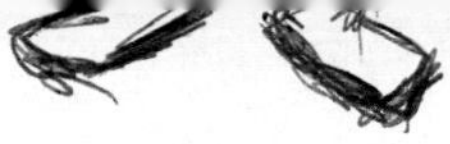

Module II

The Genetics of IDD:
Syndromes and Phenotypes

Pre-test

Module II: The Genetics of IDD: Syndromes and Phenotypes

_____ 1. Among the causes of intellectual/developmental disabilities are:
(a) Chromosomal abnormalities
(b) No known causes
(c) Exposure to toxins
(d) All of the above

_____ 2. True or false: Deletions and duplications of chromosomes along a DNA strand are quite common and collectively account for a significant minority of genetic causes of intellectual disability.

_____ 3. The specific and characteristic repertoire exhibited by people with a genetic disorder best describes:
(a) Genetic phenotype
(b) Behavioral phenotype
(c) Chromosomal abnormality
(d) The behavior of black holes approaching a vacuum

_____ 4. There are many benefits of genetic testing, but this is not considered one of them:
(a) Identification of a specific syndrome that may have associated medical vulnerabilities and behavioral phenotypes or specific behavioral patterns
(b) Early diagnosis assists with early identification of strengths
(c) Identification of which parent has contributed the chromosomes causing the abnormality
(d) Preventative health care for medical vulnerabilities

_____ 5. True or False: Recent studies indicate there are epigenetic changes associated with FASD.

_____ 6. Of the following, which are considered to be medical vulnerabilities associated with Down syndrome:
(a) Congenital heart defects
(b) Respiratory and hearing problems
(c) Thyroid conditions
(d) Childhood leukemia
(e) All of the above
(f) None of the above

_____ 7. Fragile X syndrome is a genetic condition that causes a range of developmental problems. Which of the following is not associated with Fragile X?
(a) Can affect males and females equally
(b) Can result in a predisposition to anxiety and hyperactive behavior
(c) About one-third of people who have Fragile X also have features of autism spectrum disorder, such as impairments with communication and social interactions
(d) Fragile X syndrome does not always cause intellectual disability, but most people who have Fragile X have a mild or moderate intellectual disability

_____ 8. People with autism spectrum disorder tend to have difficulty with:
(a) Social disinhibition
(b) Weight control
(c) Communication/language
(d) Impulsiveness

_____ 9. The behavioral phenotype of Angelman syndrome is characterized by each of the following except:
(a) A happy demeanor with prominent "smiling"
(b) Repeated self-injury
(c) General exuberance associated with hypermotive behavior
(d) Reduced behavioral adaptive skills
(e) A full range of emotions (prominent smiling is potentially a motor reaction to physical or mental stimuli)

_____ 10. True or false: Treatment of ASD usually focuses around early intervention with proper medical care, education/behavior therapy, language and speech therapy, occupational therapy and physical therapy.

MODULE 2

Slide 1

Module II

The Genetics of IDD:
Syndromes and Phenotypes

Slide 2

Learning Objectives

- Describe the many causes of IDD and identify five common syndromes.
- Describe what is meant by "behavioral phenotype."
- Understand the benefit of genetic testing and knowing the cause of the genetic disorder.

Slide 3

There are thousands of potential causes of intellectual/developmental disability. Among them:

- Chromosomal abnormalities
- Environmental genetic abnormalities
- Infections
- Metabolic issues/disorders
- Nutritional deficiencies/abnormalities
- Toxicity
- Trauma (prenatal and perinatal)
- Unknown

Whitaker, 2014

Slide 4

Advances in genetics over the past 30 years have lead to identification of previously unknown causes of intellectual/developmental disabilities. As a result, the number of identified genetic causes of IDD has grown exponentially into the thousands.

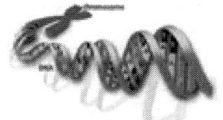

Deciphering Developmental Disorders, 2015

Slide 5

Syndromes

A syndrome is a disease or disorder that has more than one identifying feature or symptom. Each particular genetic syndrome will have many typical, common features, depending on which aspects of development are affected by the abnormal genes or chromosomes.

Slide 6

Advances in Genetic Testing

The study of genetics was advanced by the work of Gregor Mendel in the mid-nineteenth century.

Significant advancements in the understanding of genetics were made in the late twentieth century, including the ability to map the human genome and perform testing that can help identify what genetic changes are responsible for various aspects of disturbances in development.

Deciphering Developmental Disorders, 2015

Slide 7

Definition of Phenotype:

The phenotype of a genetic syndrome is the set of physical characteristics produced by a genetic abnormality or genotype.

Definition of Behavioral Phenotype:

The specific and characteristic repertoire exhibited by people with a genetic disorder.

Slide 8

Behavioral Phenotypes

- Are not set in stone
- Look at syndromes rather than set diagnoses
- Behavioral manifestations arise from the interaction of genes and environment
- Present a wide range of symptoms
- Used as clues, not as expectations

Watson & Griffiths, 2016

Slide 9

The Importance of Genetic Testing

Genetic testing can lead to identification of a specific syndrome that may have associated

- Medical vulnerabilities
- Behavioral phenotypes or specific behavioral patterns

Watson & Griffiths, 2016

Slide 10

8 Benefits of Syndrome Identification

1. Increased understanding of mental health risks and development of resilience.
2. Cross-discipline collaboration to develop more effective treatment strategies.
3. Increased attention to understanding people from a bio-psycho-social perspective.
4. Allows people to make informed decisions about reproductive choices.
5. Increased support for families, care providers, and the person.
6. Along with challenges, early diagnosis allows early identification of strengths.
7. Early identification of learning challenges and educational adaptations.
8. Preventative health care.

Watson & Griffiths, 2016

Slide 11

Common Types of Intellectual Developmental Disability

- Down syndrome
- Fragile X syndrome
- Prader-Willi syndrome
- Williams syndrome
- Smith-Magenis syndrome
- 22q11.2 deletion syndrome
- Angelman syndrome
- Smith-Lemli-Opitz syndrome
- Autism Spectrum Disorders (ASD)
- Fetal Alcohol Spectrum Disorder (FASD)

DM-ID 2, 2016

Slide 12

Down Syndrome

Down syndrome is a genetic condition causing a set of delays in physical and intellectual development as a result of having an extra copy of chromosome 21.

All people with Down syndrome experience cognitive delays, but the effect is usually mild to moderate.

National Down Syndrome Society (NDSS, 2012)

MODULE 2

Slide 13

People who have Down syndrome have increased risk for certain medical conditions such as:

- congenital heart defects
- respiratory and hearing problems
- Alzheimer's disease
- childhood leukemia
- thyroid conditions

A few of the common physical traits of Down syndrome are low muscle tone, small stature, an upward slant to the eyes and a single deep crease across the center of the palm.

CDC, 2018

Slide 14

Down Syndrome Phenotype

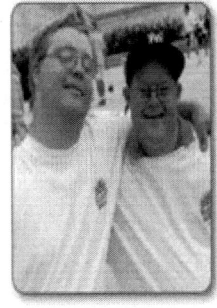

People who have Down syndrome typically have a smaller-than-average head, upward-slanting eyes, a broad neck and a tendency toward obesity.

DM-ID-2, 2016

Slide 15

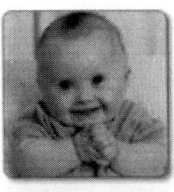
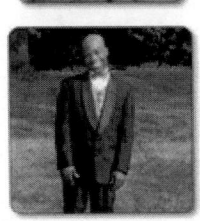

Behavioral Phenotypes
Down Syndrome

- Tendency to be noncompliant with requests
- Single-minded and tenacious
- Inattentive
- Overactive
- Argumentative
- Withdrawn
- Predisposition to depression and dementia among adults
- ADHD

Slide 16

Fragile X Syndrome

- Fragile X syndrome is a genetic condition that causes a range of developmental problems, including learning disabilities and cognitive impairment.
- Usually males are more severely affected by this disorder than females.
- Fragile X syndrome does not always cause intellectual disability, but most people who have Fragile X have a mild or moderate intellectual disability.

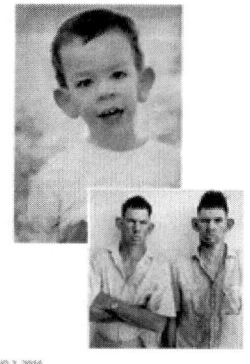

DM-ID, 2007

Slide 17

Fragile X Phenotype

People who have Fragile X often have common physical features such as:
- A long face
- Prominent ears
- High arched palate
- Flat feet
- Soft skin
- Other connective tissue abnormalities

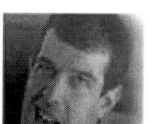

DM-ID 2, 2016

Slide 18

Behavioral Phenotypes Fragile X Syndrome

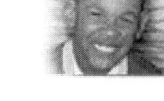

- Social anxiety
- Shyness
- Gaze aversion
- Perseveration
- Autism/PDD
- Inattention, hyperactivity, sadness or depression (primarily females)
- Attention Deficit Disorder

Dykens et al., 2000

Slide 19

Prader-Willi Syndrome

Prader-Willi syndrome (PWS) is a genetic disorder that is complex in origin but results from an abnormality of the 15th chromosome.

PWS causes a wide range of development problems including learning disabilities and cognitive impairment.

The genetic mutation that causes PWS generally occurs randomly but can be heritable.

Slide 20

Prader-Willi Syndrome Phenotype

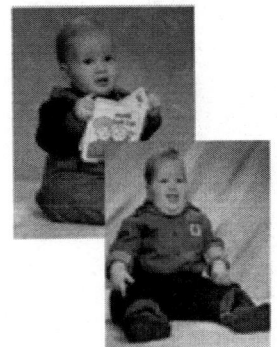

People who have PWS typically share common physical features including:
- short in stature
- hyperphagia
- obesity
- small hands and feet
- dysmorphic facial features
- hypogonadism
- low muscle tone

Slide 21

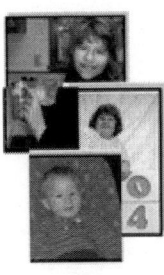

Behavioral Phenotypes Prader-Willi Syndrome

The behavioral phenotypes of Prader-Willi syndrome include:
- Non-food obsessions & compulsions
- Skin-picking
- Temper tantrums (emotional and
- Physical outbursts for adults)
- Perseveration
- Willfulness
- Underactivity
- OCD
- Mood disorders

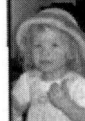

Dykens Hodapp & Finucane, 2000

Slide 22

Williams Syndrome

Williams syndrome is a genetically caused neurodevelopmental disorder that results in a wide variety of health, developmental and cognitive challenges.

It is caused by the deletion of genetic material from a specific region on chromosome 7.

Most people with Williams syndrome probably will have a mild to moderate intellectual disability or learning challenges. It is also characterized by a distinct personality profile.

DM-ID 2, 2016

Slide 23

Williams Syndrome
Phenotype

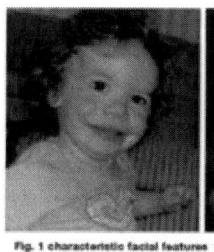 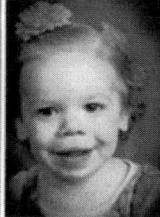

- Full lips
- Puffy cheeks
- Small jaw
- Short stature
- Spinal curvature
- Slumped posture

Fig. 1 characteristic facial features of Williams Syndrome include puffiness around the eyes, short nose, wide mouth, full lips, full cheeks and a small chin

DM-ID 2, 2016

Slide 24

Behavioral Phenotypes
Williams Syndrome

Williams syndrome has the associated behavior phenotype:
- Anxiety
- Fears
- Phobias
- Inattention
- Hyperactivity
- Social disinhibition/overly friendly
- Indiscriminate relating
- Attention Deficit Disorder

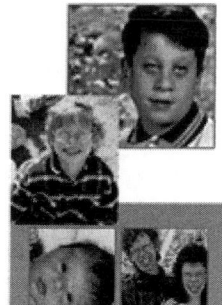

DM-ID 2, 2016

Slide 25

Smith-Magenis Syndrome

Smith-Magenis syndrome is a genetic condition causing a set of delays in physical and intellectual development as a result of a chromosome deletion.

DM-ID 2, 2016

Slide 26

Smith-Magenis Syndrome

All people with Smith-Magenis syndrome will have an intellectual disability, most commonly in the mild to moderate range.

However, there is also a predisposition to strength in:
- Long-term memory for places, things and people
- Letter/word recognition
- Simultaneous processing skills

DM-ID 2, 2016

Slide 27

Smith-Magenis Syndrome Phenotype

A person who has Smith-Magenis syndrome is likely to have:

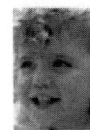

- A broad, square-shaped face with deep-set eyes
- Full cheeks
- A prominent lower jaw
- The appearance of flattened middle of the face and bridge of the nose
- Mouth will tend to turn downward
- Full, outward-curving upper lip
- Dental abnormalities are common

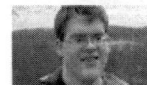

Poisson, et al, 2015

Slide 28

Behavioral Phenotypes
Smith-Magenis Syndrome

The chromosome deletion responsible for Smith-Magenis syndrome also results in a behavioral phenotype.

Common behavioral challenges can include:

- Self-injury
- Aggression
- Anxiety
- Impulsiveness
- Difficulty paying attention

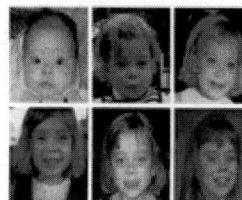

Slide 29

22q11.2 Deletion Syndrome

22q11.2 Deletion syndrome is genetic disorder that can lead to a wide variety of physical and developmental delays. Features can vary widely, even in members of the same family.

22q11.2 Deletion syndrome can cause mild to moderate intellectual disability and causes a predisposition to mental health problems, particularly in adulthood.

Bassett, & Chow, 1999

Slide 30

22q11.2 Deletion Syndrome

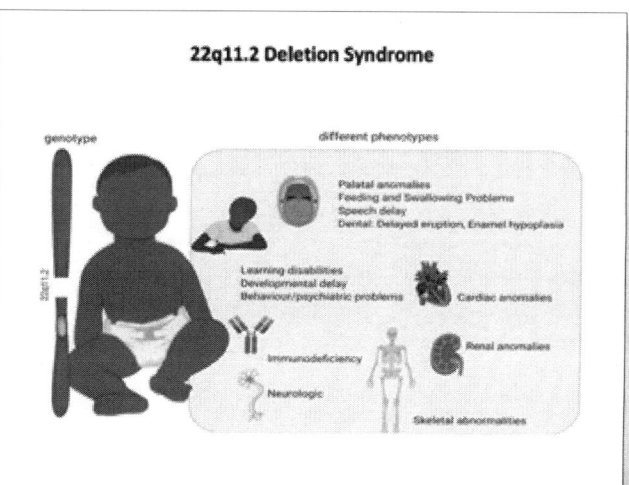

Slide 31

22Q Deletion Syndrome
Phenotype

22q11.2 Deletion syndrome is associated with a number of physiological and physical differences including:

- Increased calcium levels
- Kidney abnormalities
- Immunodeficiency
- Problematic thyroid function
- Congenital heart defects
- Low platelet counts
- Velopharyngeal insufficiency (failure of palate to meet the throat during crying, swallowing and speech)
- Underdeveloped chin
- Low-set ears

Slide 32

Behavioral Phenotypes
22q11.2 Deletion Syndrome

There are several common behavioral challenges observed in people who have 22q11.2 Deletion syndrome, including:

- Overactivity
- Impulsivity
- Emotional lability
- Shyness
- Withdrawal
- Disinhibition
- Immaturity
- Self-talk
- Anger issues
- Anxiety

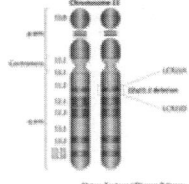

Mikhail et al, 2914   McDonald-McGinn et al, 2015

Slide 33

Angelman Syndrome

Angelman syndrome (AS) is a genetic disorder that primarily affects the nervous system in a number of ways, including:

- Delayed development
- Severe speech impairment
- Ataxia (movement and balance problems)
- Microcephaly (in most cases)
- Epilepsy (in most cases)

It can be caused by a deletion, mutation or replication error in a portion of chromosome 15 or a mutation in the gene UBE3A.

AS causes a full range of intellectual/developmental disabilities.

Slide 34

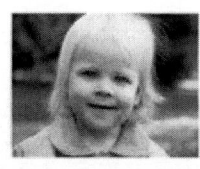

**Angelman Syndrome
Phenotype**

- Hair, skin and eyes that are light in color (hypopigmentation)
- Scoliosis is common
- As children, appear thin with low or near-normal subcutaneous fat

Slide 35

Behavioral Phenotype Angelman Syndrome

Characterized by:

- A happy demeanor with prominent "smiling"
- Poorly specific laughing
- General exuberance associated with hypermotive behavior
- Reduced behavioral adaptive skills

Cassidy & Allanson, 2010

Slide 36

Smith-Lemli-Opitz Syndrome

Smith-Lemli-Opitz syndrome is a genetic disorder that causes intellectual/developmental disability and a range of physical problems.

It is characterized by distinctive physical, intellectual and behavioral characteristics.

Smith-Lemli-Opitz syndrome is caused by a mutation on the gene that is responsible for the activity of a cholesterol reductase and prevents cells from producing enough cholesterol.

Cassidy & Allanson, 2010

Slide 37

Smith-Lemli-Opitz
Phenotype

- Growth delay
- Microcephaly
- Extra fingers and toes
- Fused second and third toes
- Cleft palate
- Underdeveloped external genitals in males
- Distinctive facial features

Slide 38

Smith-Lemli-Opitz
Behavioral Phenotype

- Repeated self-injury
- Prolonged temper tantrums
- Violent outbursts
- Hyperactivity

(Bianconi, Cross, Wassif, & Porter, 2015)

Slide 39

Autism Spectrum Disorder

Autism Spectrum Disorder (ASD) is a complex condition that impacts normal brain development and affects a person's social relationships, communication, interests and behavior across multiple contexts. ASD is a single condition with different levels of symptom severity.

DSM 5, 2013

Slide 40

Slide 41

Autism Spectrum Disorder

ASD is characterized by:

- Persistent deficits in social communication and social interaction across multiple contexts
- Restricted, repetitive patterns of behavior, interests or activities

DSM 5, 2013

Slide 42

Autism Spectrum Disorder

ASD is typically noticed in the first or second year of life with:

- Delay or abnormality in language and play.
- Repetitive behaviors, such as spinning things or lining up small objects.
- Unusual interests, such as preoccupations with stop signs or ceiling fans.

DiCicco-Bloom et al., 2006

M
O
D
U
L
E

2

Slide 43

Autism Spectrum Disorder
Phenotype

People who have autism spectrum disorders often have difficulties with:

- Abnormal responses to sensory stimulation
- Behavior problems
- Variability of intellectual functioning
- Uneven development profile
- Difficulties in sleeping, toileting and eating
- Immune irregularities
- Nutritional deficiencies
- Gastrointestinal problems

McCray, Trevvett, & Frost, 2014)

Slide 44

Autism Spectrum Disorder
Behavioral Phenotype

Deficits in social interaction can be observed in these areas:

- Failure to initiate or sustain conversations (e.g., turn-taking)
- Serious deficits in the ability to make friendships
- Failure to respond to their names when called
- Appearing not to listen when spoken to
- Difficulty identifying boundaries of others

McEvoy, Rogers, and Pennington, 2006

Slide 45

Autism Spectrum Disorder
Behavioral Phenotype

Restricted repetitive behaviors, interests and activities may be observed as:

- Perseveration of interests and activities—people who have ASD typically have a narrow range of interests
- Repetitive, stereotyped body movements such as hand-flicking, spinning or rocking
- Perseverations might extend to food
- Dependence on routine

McEvoy, Rogers & Pennington, 2006

Slide 46

Fetal Alcohol Spectrum Disorder
(FASD)

FASD is a term used to describe a range of disabilities caused by prenatal exposure to alcohol.

While each person impacted by FASD is unique, brain damage typically results in various symptoms commonly observed in people who have an FASD.

Astley, 2004

Slide 47

FASD Phenotype

FASD is associated with several potential physical features and challenges that can include:
- Low birth weight and trouble gaining weight
- Smaller-than-average head circumference
- Heart defects
- Anomalies to ears, eyes, liver and joints

Facial features associated with FASD will occur only if there was exposure to alcohol during a specific period of pregnancy. The features are:

- Small eye openings
- Smooth, wide philtrum
- Thin upper lip

Astley et al, 2002

Slide 48

FASD Behavioral Phenotype

People with FASD often share common behavioral traits, including:
- Memory problems
- Difficulty storing and retrieving information
- Inconsistent performance ("on" and "off") days
- Impulsivity, distractibility, disorganization
- Ability to repeat instructions, but inability to put them into action
- Difficulty with abstractions, such as math, money management, time concepts
- Cognitive processing deficits (may think more slowly)
- Slow auditory pace (may only understand every third word of a normally paced conversation)
- Developmental lags (may act younger than chronological age)
- Inability to predict outcomes or understand consequence

McHugh/FAS Center, 2001

Slide 49

FASD

Preventable *Secondary* Characteristics

In the absence of accurate diagnosis, patterns of defensive behaviors commonly develop over time. These are called secondary characteristics of FASD:

- Fatigue, tantrums
- Irritability, frustration, anger, aggression
- Fear, anxiety, avoidance, withdrawal
- Shutdown, lying, running away
- Trouble at home, school and community
- Legal trouble
- Drug/alcohol abuse
- Mental health problems (depression, self-injury, suicidal tendencies)

Streissguth et al., 2004

MODULE 2

Post-test

Module II: The Genetics of IDD: Syndromes and Phenotypes

_____ 1. Among the causes of intellectual/developmental disabilities are:
(a) Chromosomal abnormalities
(b) No known causes
(c) Exposure to toxins
(d) All of the above

_____ 2. True or false: Deletions and duplications of chromosomes along a DNA strand are quite common and collectively account for a significant minority of genetic causes of intellectual disability.

_____ 3. The specific and characteristic repertoire exhibited by people with a genetic disorder best describes:
(a) Genetic phenotype
(b) Behavioral phenotype
(c) Chromosomal abnormality
(d) The behavior of black holes approaching a vacuum

_____ 4. There are many benefits of genetic testing, but this is not considered one of them:
(a) Identification of a specific syndrome that may have associated medical vulnerabilities and behavioral phenotypes or specific behavioral patterns
(b) Early diagnosis assists with early identification of strengths
(c) Identification of which parent has contributed the chromosomes causing the abnormality
(d) Preventative health care for medical vulnerabilities

_____ 5. True or False: Recent studies indicate there are epigenetic changes associated with FASD.

_____ 6. Of the following, which are considered to be medical vulnerabilities associated with Down syndrome:
(a) Congenital heart defects
(b) Respiratory and hearing problems
(c) Thyroid conditions
(d) Childhood leukemia
(e) All of the above
(f) None of the above

M
O
D
U
L
E

2

_____ 7. Fragile X syndrome is a genetic condition that causes a range of developmental problems. Which of the following is not associated with Fragile X?

(a) Can affect males and females equally

(b) Can result in a predisposition to anxiety and hyperactive behavior

(c) About one-third of people who have Fragile X also have features of autism spectrum disorder, such as impairments with communication and social interactions

(d) Fragile X syndrome does not always cause intellectual disability, but most people who have Fragile X have a mild or moderate intellectual disability

_____ 8. People with autism spectrum disorder tend to have difficulty with:

(a) Social disinhibition

(b) Weight control

(c) Communication/language

(d) Impulsiveness

_____ 9. The behavioral phenotype of Angelman syndrome is characterized by each of the following except:

(a) A happy demeanor with prominent "smiling"

(b) Repeated self-injury

(c) General exuberance associated with hypermotive behavior

(d) Reduced behavioral adaptive skills

(e) A full range of emotions (prominent smiling is potentially a motor reaction to physical or mental stimuli)

_____ 10. True or false: Treatment of ASD usually focuses around early intervention with proper medical care, education/behavior therapy, language and speech therapy, occupational therapy and physical therapy.

MODULE 2

Supplemental Materials

Module II: The Genetics of IDD: Syndromes and Phenotypes

The study of human genetics can help us understand more about human nature, health, diseases, effective treatments and the general nature of human life. Humans are *diploid* organisms, meaning we get one set of genes (called *alleles*) from each biological parent.

The combination of these pairs of genes is called your *genotype*. The genotype determines the actual traits that people have (traits are called the phenotypes), such as eye color, nearsightedness and whether or not someone can roll their tongue, for example.

There are a number of human traits that can be linked to different types of genetic hereditary patterns. The following is a list of observable human traits. Think about your own traits or phenotype. Do you know if either of your biological parents shares these traits?

Dominant	Recessive
Widow's peak	Straight hairline
Facial dimples	No facial dimples
Unattached (free) earlobe	Attached earlobe
Cleft chin	Smooth chin
Ability to roll tongue*	No ability to roll tongue
Extra finger or toe	Five fingers and toes
Straight thumb	Hitchhiker's thumb
Freckles	No freckles
Roman nose	No prominent bridge
Photic sneeze reflex (Achoo syndrome)**	No Achoo reflex
Hand clasping: left thumb on top***	Hand clasping: right thumb on top

*Tongue rolling: If you have the ability to roll the sides of your tongue upward to form a closed tube, you have the dominant phenotype for this motor skill. Those who are not dominant for this trait cannot roll their tongue, no matter how hard they may try.

**Achoo syndrome: This dominant trait is also called the photo sneeze reflex. If, when suddenly exposed to light, you sneeze (usually two or three times), you have the genes for Achoo syndrome. Next time you go to a movie, exit the dark theater through a door that leads directly outside. It's fun to wait outside and watch the people emerge from the movie. Some will sneeze as soon as they are exposed to light.

***Hand clasping: Clasp your hands together (without thinking about it!). Most people place their left thumb on top of their right, and this happens to be the dominant phenotype. Now try clasping your hands so the opposite thumb is on top. It may feel strange and uncomfortable.

Other observable genetic traits are detached/attached earlobes, pronounced bend in the thumb (hitchhiker's thumb) and widow's peak (a V-shaped point in the hairline in the center of the forehead). Visual representations of many traits can be found at https://learn.genetics.utah.edu/content/basics/observable/

Can you think of other traits that might be shared by your biological relatives? Curly hair? Eye color?

_____

_____

_____

Genetic Assessment of Adults with Intellectual and Developmental Disabilities: Frequently Asked Questions

Many adults whose intellectual and developmental disabilities (IDD) are of unknown origin may benefit from etiologic assessment or reassessment. Etiologic assessment is often helpful in planning preventive care, treatment, and management strategies.

The information sheet at the link below answers common questions that family physicians may have about including genetic testing professionals involved in their patients' care. It provides information for finding the nearest Canadian genetic center, indications for referral and how to make a referral, and outlines information to give the person with an intellectual and developmental disability and their support persons regarding the referral process.

https://ddprimarycare.surreyplace.ca/wp-content/uploads/2019/05/2.1-Genetic-Assessment_may-27.pdf

1. **Why might a genetic assessment be helpful?**
    Optimal medical management: It may be possible to develop a tailored medical and psychosocial management approach to address physical and mental health issues once the etiology is established. For example, people with Down syndrome have an increased probability of developing thyroid disease throughout their lifespan and will benefit from earlier and more regular screening than guidelines for the general population recommend.

    Identifying a genetic etiology can have health management consequences for family members. For example, in the Fragile X syndrome, pre-mutation carrier males and females have the potential to develop Fragile X-associated tremor/ataxia syndrome and females have an increased risk of premature ovarian insufficiency.

Family reasons: The patient and other family members may want information about the cause of the IDD and the risk of recurrence within the family. There can be substantial guilt about having a child with IDD. Knowing the cause can relieve parental guilt and provide reassurance. As well, with this knowledge, family members may be able to find support by connecting with syndrome-specific organizations.

2. **Which diagnoses can be detected through genetic testing?**
   Over 2,500 genes have been associated with syndromic and non-syndromic IDD, including autism spectrum disorder. This number is continuing to increase as our knowledge expands.

   Genetic tests can identify single gene pathogenic variants (mutations), whole or partial chromosome duplications and deletions (including microduplications and microdeletions), imprinting defects, and mitochondrial disorders.

   Relevant to the population with IDD, examples of diagnoses from genetic testing include Down syndrome, Fragile X syndrome, Prader-Willi syndrome, Williams syndrome, Smith-Magenis syndrome and 22q11.2 deletion syndrome. Some syndrome-specific reviews are available at Gene Reviews, University of Washington (www.genereviews.org).

Reference: Genetic Assessment of Adults with Intellectual and Developmental Disabilities: Frequently Asked Questions. Forster-Gibson, C., Developmental Disabilities Primary Care Program of Surrey Place, Toronto, 2019.

Surrey Place Centre Health Watch Tables

Health Watch Tables offer information on a variety of syndromes and their related health concerns. These tables were created to complement Canadian guidelines on caring for adults with intellectual and developmental disabilities

Health Watch Tables are available for:

- Down syndrome
- Fragile X syndrome
- Prader-Willi syndrome
- Smith-Magenis syndrome
- 22q11.2 deletion syndrome
- Fetal alcohol spectrum disorder
- Williams syndrome

MODULE 2

- Autism spectrum disorder
- Angelman syndrome

Find the Health Watch Tables here: https://ddprimarycare.surreyplace.ca/tools-2/health-watch-tables/

MODULE 2

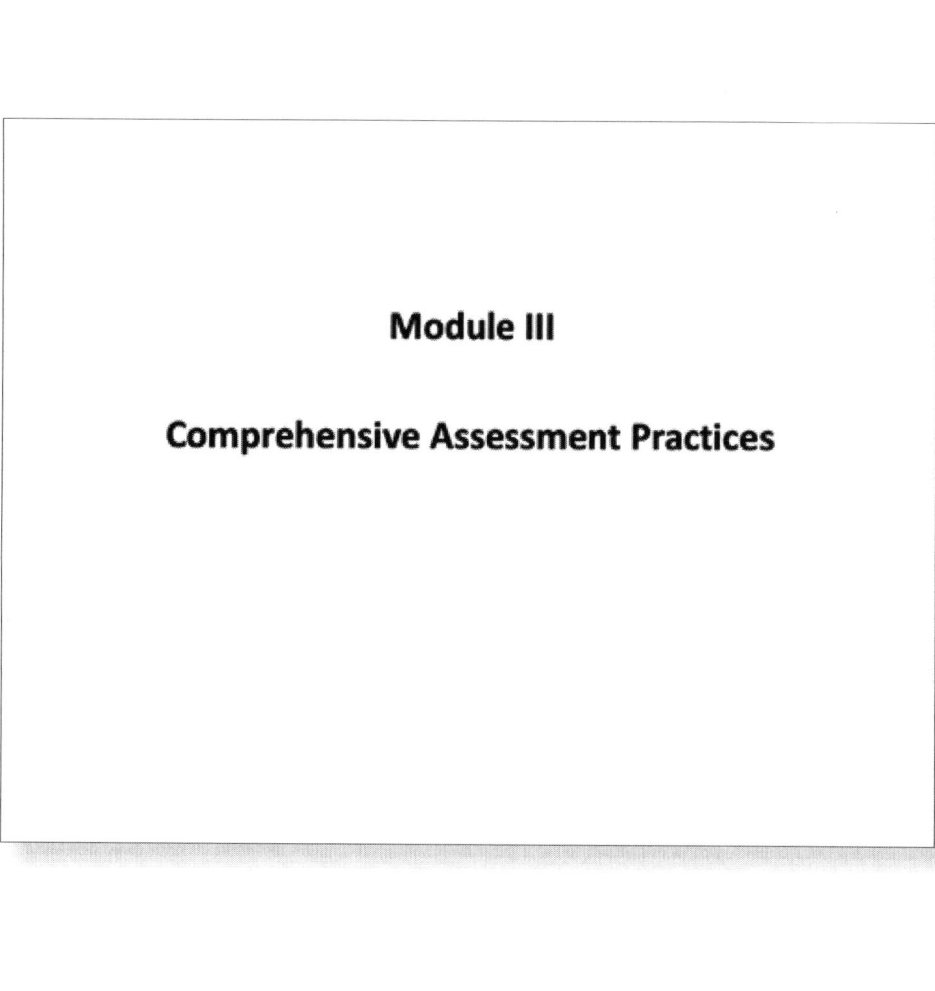

Module III

Comprehensive Assessment Practices

Pre-test

Module III: Comprehensive Assessment Practices

_____ 1.   Which model is the most clinically useful in identifying the nature of challenging behavior in persons with IDD?
(a) Medical Model
(b) Communication Model
(c) Behavior Model
(d) Integrative Model

_____ 2.   Possible functions of challenging behavior in people with IDD/MI can include:
(a) To gain attention from others
(b) To escape or avoid demands
(c) To obtain tangible items or opportunities
(d) All of the above

_____ 3.   Best practice in assessment and diagnosis for people with IDD/MI refers to:
(a) The Bio-psycho-social model
(b) Behavior analysis
(c) Mental health assessments
(d) An annual physical completed by a health professional

_____ 4.   One of the first steps to completing a functional assessment is:
(a) Describing the target behavior; assigning an operational definition
(b) Understanding the behavior from the perspective of the person who directly observes it and the problem it causes for other people
(c) Identifying the patterns of triggers to help figure out how a behavior is maintained
(d) Assessing the effectiveness of different approaches on the target behavior

_____ 5.   Which of the following is the most suggestive indicator that a behavior pattern may be the result of a mental illness:
(a) The behavior is exhibited only at home
(b) The behavior occurs in all environments; it is not observed just in specific settings
(c) The behavior never occurs when the person's favorite direct support professional is supporting him/her
(d) The person appears to be able to start and stop the behavior at will

_____ 6.   The bio-psycho-social model _____
(a) Does not require the review of existing data or background information to contribute to

the assessment process

(b) Recognizes that mental health is defined only by the relative absence of psychological distress

(c) Incorporates the effects of biomedical and psychological factors and how these influences interrelate

(d) Recognizes that the clinical interview can be completed by reviewing the documented history and reports compiled about the person

_____ 7. Which of the following statements is accurate?
(a) Medical problems in people with IDD are easily recognized
(b) Dental problems in people with IDD are easily recognized
(c) Rapid onset in a change in behavior patterns is likely because behavioral problems are directly associated with having the condition of IDD
(d) Causes of self-injurious behavior in people with IDD can be related to an underlying medical condition

_____ 8. True or false: In addition to the client's health history (medical, psychological, substance use), clinicians should obtain the health history of family members.

_____ 9. True or false: People with IDD experience the full range of psychiatric disorders as compared to the general population.

_____ 10. Medical conditions:
(a) Can be present when behavioral problems are exhibited
(b) Are often underdiagnosed
(c) Can be masked as behavioral problems
(d) All of the above

M
O
D
U
L
E

3

Slide 1

Module III

Comprehensive Assessment Practices

Slide 2

This module includes content related to conceptual models related to behavior problems: integrative approach, functional assessment of behavior and assessment and diagnostic practices.

Slide 3

Learning Objectives

- Articulate the elements of behavioral, medical, communication and physical models of problem behavior.
- List the components and importance of the Integrative Model.
- Articulate the importance of medical assessments in the assessment process.

Slide 4

**Conceptual Models Related to
Behavioral Problems:**

An Integrated Assessment Approach

Slide 5

Five Conceptual Models:

1. Medical Model

2. Communication Model

3. Behavioral Model

4. Psychiatric Model

5. Integrative Model (1-4)

Fletcher et al. (2016)

Slide 6

1. **Medical Model**

- Problem behaviors are exhibited because of coexisting medical problems

- Assessment of potential medical problems involves conducting a full medical workup

- Treatment focuses on addressing the underlying medical problem

Engel, 1977

Slide 7

2. Communication Model

- Views behavioral problems as reflecting "challenging behaviors" in persons who have deficits in language skills.

- Treatment—teach communication skills.

- Assessment focuses on evaluation of skills, deficits and communicative intent.

McClintock, Hall & Oliver, 2003

Slide 8

3. Behavioral Model

- Problem behaviors are viewed according to learning principles

- Assessment identifies the antecedent and consequences of the problematic behavior

- Treatment focuses on changing or eliminating behavior though behavioral approaches

- Does not usually identify people's needs/emotions

Baer, Wolf & Risley, 1968

Slide 9

4. Psychiatric Model

- Views problem behavior as a possible manifestation of a mental disorder

- Presentation of problem behaviors may be associated with a psychiatric disorder

- Assessment based on a bio-psycho-social model

- Treatment focuses on underlying psychiatric disorders

Engel, 1977

MODULE 3

Slide 10

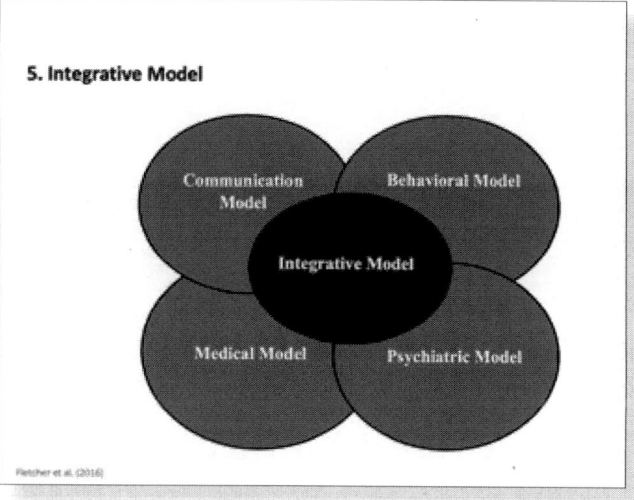

5. Integrative Model

Communication Model

Behavioral Model

Integrative Model

Medical Model

Psychiatric Model

Fletcher et al. (2016)

Slide 11

The Relationship of Challenging Behavior and IDD

Type of Model	Medical	Communication	Behavioral	Psychiatric
Assessment	Medical evaluation by primary care physician	Standardized administered measure of expressive language	Functional Analysis	DM-ID
Problem Identification	Constipation	Speech and language impairment	Function/ need being met through behavior	Affective disorder, mania
Treatment	Medication for bowel movement (laxative)	Functional communication skill training	Addressing unmet need, supporting appropriate behavior	Medication treatment, psychotherapy

Fletcher et al. (2016)

Slide 12

Case Vignette: John

- 15-year-old male, IQ = 50
- living with parents
- becoming angry/hostile at school with other students
- recent onset of behavioral problems:
  - SIB
  - property destruction
- sleep disturbance
- displays agitation and aggression
- limited verbal communication skills
- appetite decreased
- constipation
- no previous psychiatric history

Fletcher et al. (2016)

Slide 13

The Function of Behavior

Behaviors may persist because the individual...

- enjoys the sensory experience — it feels better, satisfies a need or impulse (internal triggers, internal rewards)
- escapes or avoids demands or things he or she doesn't like to do
- gains attention from others
- obtains tangible items or opportunities — access to something he or she prefers

Beavers, Iwata & Lerman, 2013

Slide 14

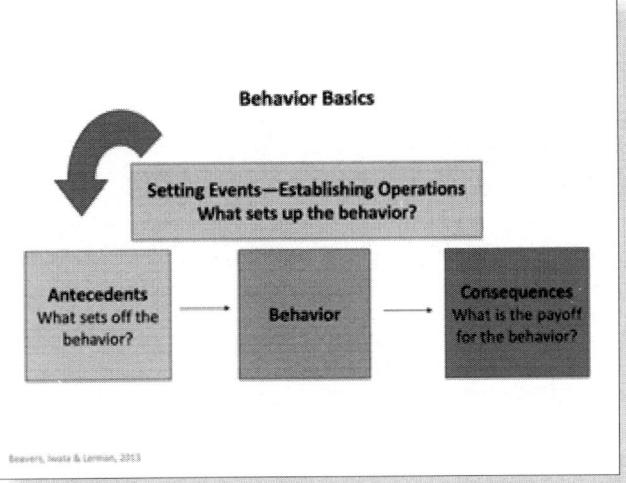

Behavior Basics

Setting Events—Establishing Operations
What sets up the behavior?

Antecedents
What sets off the behavior? → **Behavior** → **Consequences**
What is the payoff for the behavior?

Beavers, Iwata & Lerman, 2013

Slide 15

Considerations of Functional Assessment

- A pattern of behavior that repeats
- Understand why the behavior occurs
  - What are the antecedents/precursors; what "sets off" the behavior?
  - Are there any setting events, things that set the person up to do the behavior?
  - What are the consequences/outcomes; what does the person get as a result?
- Is the behavior:
  - an attempt to communicate?
  - a way to avoid or obtain something?
  - the result of a medical condition or other factor?

Iwata et al., 1994

Slide 16

The Steps to a Functional Assessment

- Describe what the target behavior is, the operational definition.
- Interview the person or care providers.
- Observe the person to see what else might be happening.
- Use the interview and observation to make some guesses about the antecedents and consequences.
- Identify antecedents, setting events and consequences (outcomes).
- Look for patterns to identify function.

Iwata et al., 1994

Slide 17

Look for Patterns

- The same type of triggers tend to set the behavior off.
- People respond in similar ways to maintain the behavior; the person gets the same kind of outcome.
- Setting events (establishing operations) make behavior more likely to occur when trigger is present.
- The behavior doesn't have to happen every time the trigger is present but work enough to make the behavior "worth it" for the individual.

Iwata et al., 1994

Slide 18

Involving Direct Support Professionals (DSPs) and Caregivers in Plan Development

- DSPs often work closest to and spend most time with people
- Encourage contributions, observations, hypotheses, ideas, intervention strategies
- DSPs can identify trends and missing puzzle pieces that managers and behaviorists often cannot
- Foster control and confidence
- Promote participation and involvement in planning
- Consider opinions and answer questions
- Provide ongoing support and guidance

Slide 19

Bio-psycho-social framework: An approach to describing and explaining how biological, psychological and social factors combine and interact to influence physical and mental health.

Psychological
- Learning
- Emotions
- Thinking
- Attitudes
- Memory
- Perceptions
- Beliefs
- Stress Management Strategies

Biological
- Genetic Predisposition
- Neurochemistry
- Effect of Medications
- Immune Response
- Fight-flight response
- Physiological responses
- HPA axis

Social
- Social Support
- Family Background
- Interpersonal Relationships
- Cultural Traditions
- Socio-economic status
- Physical exercise
- Biofeedback   Poverty
- Medical Care

Adapted from Griffiths & Gardner, 2002

Slide 20

The Bio-Psycho-Social Model

- Incorporates the effects of biomedical and psychological factors and how these influences interrelate.
- Uses assessment information to guide selection of diagnostically based interventions.

Griffiths & Gardner 2002

Slide 21

The Bio-Psycho-Social Model

- Identifies skills and related supports required by the individual to cope effectively with multiple bio-psycho-social influences.
- Is proactive in focus.
- Provides for translation of multiple modalities of influence in a common model.

Griffiths & Gardner 2002

MODULE 3

Slide 22

The Bio-Psycho-Social Model

- Provides an integrated multimodal treatment plan.
- Recognizes that mental health consists of both the presence of personal contentment and the relative absence of psychological distress.

Griffiths & Gardner 2002

Slide 23

A comprehensive assessment includes:

1. Reviewing reports
2. Interviewing family
3. Interviewing care provider/DSP
4. Completing direct observation
5. Conducting a clinical interview

Morrison & Gillig, 2012

Slide 24

A comprehensive assessment includes:

- Obtain records in advance
    - School, medical, development and family
- Become familiar with collateral informants who attend the interview
    - Parents, care provider, service coordinators
- Understand that the assessment interview can be stressful for all involved
    - Interviewer will need to be alert for increased distress on part of the client

Morrison & Gillig, 2002

M
O
D
U
L
E

3

Slide 25

- Assessment interview probably will take more time than with a neurotypical person
- Examiner needs to use language that correlates with the expressive and receptive language skills of the client
    - Simple language
    - Reflection
    - Stay away from abstract concepts and analogies

Morrison & Gillig, 2012

Slide 26

Important components of a mental health assessment:

- Watch for signs the person is trying to respond to questions in a way that will please the interviewer.
- Parroting and perseverating habits may interfere with the accuracy of the responses.
- Multiple assessment interviews may be needed to obtain a full assessment.

Morrison & Gillig, 2012

Slide 27

Historical Data Gathering
- Source of information and reason for referral
- History of presenting problem and past psychiatric history
- Family health history
- Social and developmental history

Fletcher et al. (2016)

Slide 28

I. Source of information and reason for referral

- Who made the referral?

- What is different from baseline behavior?

- Why make the referral now?

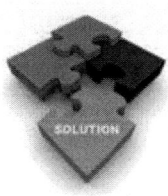

Fletcher et al. (2016)

Slide 29

II. History of presenting problem and past psychiatric history

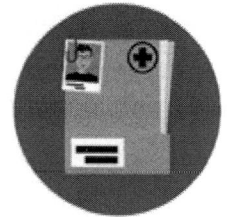

- How long has the problem occurred?
- History of mental health treatment
- Trauma history

Fletcher et al. (2016)

Slide 30

III. Personal and family health history

- Medical, psychiatric and substance abuse history
- Psychotropic medications
- Medical conditions
- Genetic disorders
- Hypo/hyperthyroid condition
- Constipation
- Epilepsy
- Diabetes
- Gastrointestinal problem

Fletcher et al. (2016)

MODULE 3

Slide 31

IV. Social/developmental history
- Developmental milestones
- Relevant school history
- Work/vocational history
- Current work/vocational status
- Legal issues
- Relevant family dynamics
- Drug/alcohol history
- Abuse history (emotional/physical/sexual)
- Trauma history

Fletcher et al. (2016)

Slide 32

Myth: Individuals with IDD Cannot Have a Verifiable Mental Health Disorder

PREMISE
Maladaptive behaviors are a function of IDD.

REALITY
The full range of psychiatric disorders can be represented in persons with IDD.

DIAGNOSTIC IMPLICATIONS
Psychiatric diagnosis can be made using the DM-ID, DSM-5 records, service providers, family input and client interview.

Adapted from Sovner & Hurley ,1989

Slide 33

8 Diagnostic Principles for Recognizing Psychiatric Disorders in People with IDD

1. People with Intellectual/Developmental Disabilities suffer from the full range of psychiatric disorders.
2. Psychiatric disorders usually present as maladaptive behavior.
3. The origin of psychopathology has multiple etiologies.

Adapted from Sovner & Hurley, 1989

Slide 34

8 Diagnostic Principles for Recognizing Psychiatric Disorders in People with IDD

4. An acute psychiatric disorder may present as an exaggeration of longstanding maladaptive behavior.
5. Maladaptive behavior rarely occurs alone.
6. The severity of the problem is not diagnostically relevant.

Adapted from Sovner 1989

Slide 35

8 Diagnostic Principles for Recognizing Psychiatric Disorders in People with IDD

7. The clinical interview alone is rarely diagnostic.
8. It is very difficult to diagnose psychotic disorders in people with very limited verbal skills.

Adapted from Sovner 1989

Slide 36

Barriers to Diagnosis and Treatment: 15 Complicating Diagnostic Factors

1. Diagnostic overshadowing
2. Problems with polypharmacy
3. Communication deficits
4. Atypical presentation of psychiatric disorders
5. Limited life experiences
6. Medical conditions
7. Acquiescence
8. Learned behavior
9. Aggression and SIB (self-injurious behavior)
10. Sensory impairment
11. Behavioral overshadowing
12. Medication masking
13. Episodic presentation
14. Division of services
15. Lack of expertise

McGilivery & Sweetland, 2011

MODULE 3

Slide 37

A Clinical Challenge

It can be difficult to distinguish whether a behavioral problem is associated with:

- A symptom of a psychiatric disorder
- A learned behavior
- A medical condition

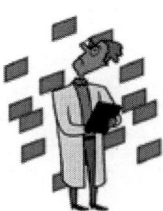

Charlot et al., 2011

Slide 38

12 Indications That a Behavioral Pattern May Be the Result of a Psychiatric Condition

1. The behavior occurs in all environments; it is not just exhibited in specific settings.

2. Behavioral strategies have been largely ineffective.

3. The individual doesn't appear to have control over their behavior. They don't appear to be able to start or stop the behavior at will.

Adapted from McGilvery & Sweetland, 2011

Slide 39

4. There are changes in sleep patterns; increased, decreased or disturbed sleep.

5. The individual is experiencing excessive mood or unusual mood patterns.

6. There are changes in the individual's appearance and a decline in their independent living skills.

Adapted from McGilvery & Sweetland,

Slide 40

7. The person may start to engage in purposeful self-harm (cutting, hitting, scratching, pulling out hair).

8. The person may start to show signs of hallucination, such as staring to the side or corners and not appear to track conversations.

9. There may be changes in eating patterns such as eating less or more.

Adapted from McGilvery & Sweetland,

Slide 41

10. The individual has a history of a psychiatric disorder that was in remission.

11. There is an acute onset of the behavior. If there is a particularly rapid onset with a significant change in mental status or cognitive functioning, rule out a possible delirium with an underlying medical cause.

12. There is an unusual change in behavior patterns, such as a significant change from baseline behavior.

Adapted from McGilvery & Sweetland, 2012

Slide 42

Medical Problems and Problem Behavior

• Why do medical causes of problem behaviors get missed?

• Why do we have to be ... Sherlock Holmes?

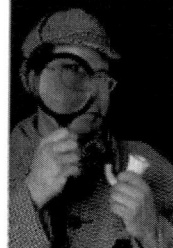

Charlot et al., 2011

Slide 43

- Medical conditions can be present when behavioral problems are exhibited.

- Medication effects/reactions can be present when behavioral problems are exhibited.

- Medical conditions are often underdiagnosed.

- Medical conditions can mask as behavioral problems.

Charlot et al., 2011

Slide 44

- Drug side effects
    - Akathisia, delirium, dyskinesia
- Endocrinological problems
    - Thyroid problems, diabetes
- Neurological problems
    - Epilepsy, other movement problems
- Other
    - Dental pain, sleep apnea, headaches, hearing and vision problems, back pain

Charlot et al., 2011

Slide 45

Group Exercise

- How do you look at potential medication side effects as part of an assessment?
- Who provides information?
- Who has expertise?

Slide 46

- Medical problems often underrecognized
- Dental problems often underrecognized
- Medical/dental problems can cause SIB
- Need to identify if there is an underlying physical problem

Charlot, et al, 2011

Slide 47

Case Example of Discomfort and SIB

- 28-year-old female with IDD referred to behavior specialist for self-injurious behavior.
- Mother noted that she scratches at her arm until it bleeds and won't leave that spot alone.
- Medical exam showed dry skin during a cold winter and recommended lotion.
- Mother subsequently reported that scratching ceased.

Slide 48

Condensed Medical Data in Chart

It is essential that all earlier medical data be available.

It is important that the past and present medical history be condensed in a format that can be easily read and placed in the person's chart.

Poindexter, 2005

M
O
D
U
L
E

3

Slide 49

Medical problems may cause significant alterations in mood and behavior that mimic acute psychiatric illness.

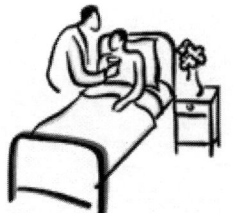

Charlot et al., 2011

Slide 50

Symptoms Reported by Informants:
Don't Confuse Phenomenology with Etiology

- MANIA
  Irritable, restless, pacing, running back and forth, can't sit still, can't focus, can't get to sleep

- AKATHISIA
  Irritable, restless, pacing, running back and forth, can't sit still, can't focus, can't get to sleep

- DEPRESSION
  Crying, won't get out of bed, decreased concentration

- CONSTIPATION
  Crying, won't get out of bed, decreased concentration

Charlot et al., 2011

Slide 51

1. Sleep Pattern:
   Quality and quantity of sleep can affect physical and mental health

   For example:
   a. Poor sleep ⇨ fatigue ⇨ irritability
   b. Depression ⇨ poor sleep ⇨ irritability
   c. Medical problem (discomfort caused by constipation) ⇨ poor sleep ⇨ irritability

   Assessment Strategy:
   Maintain sleep data.

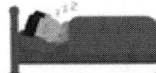

Charlot et al., 2011

M O D U L E 3

Slide 52

2. Appetite pattern:

Changes in appetite can be clues in the assessment of mental health or physical problem.

Significant weight change may indicate a medical or mental health problem.

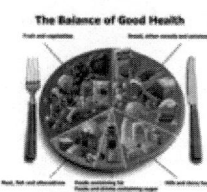

Assessment strategy:

Monitor and document a person's weight on a weekly basis.

Charlet et al., 2011

Slide 53

3. Activity level:

Activity level refers to the things a person usually does during the day. For example:

- going to work
- completing chores
- leisure time pursuits

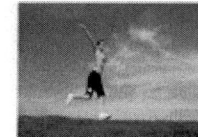

Assessment strategy:

If a person's activity level changes drastically, it may be an unrecognized medical or mental health problem.

Charlet et al., 2011

Slide 54

3. Activity level (continued):

Examples:

Arthritis ⇨ decreased activity ⇨ refuses to go to work ⇨ could be viewed as non-compliant

Depression ⇨ decreased activity ⇨ refuses to go to work ⇨ could be viewed as noncompliant

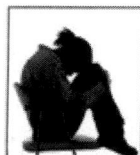

Charlet et al., 2011

Slide 55

BEAMS

- Are there any changes in the current conditions?
- Are there any changes in:
    - B = behavior
    - E = energy level*
    - A = appetite
    - M = mood
    - S = sleep patterns
- How long have the symptoms/changes been occurring?
- Is there anything that appears to help the person feel better when these signs are present?
- In what context have these changes occurred?

MODULE 3

Post-test

Module III: Comprehensive Assessment Practices

_____ 1. Which model is the most clinically useful in identifying the nature of challenging behavior in persons with IDD?
(a) Medical Model
(b) Communication Model
(c) Behavior Model
(d) Integrative Model

_____ 2. Possible functions of challenging behavior in people with IDD/MI can include:
(a) To gain attention from others
(b) To escape or avoid demands
(c) To obtain tangible items or opportunities
(d) All of the above

_____ 3. Best practice in assessment and diagnosis for people with IDD/MI refers to:
(a) The Bio-psycho-social model
(b) Behavior analysis
(c) Mental health assessments
(d) An annual physical completed by a health professional

_____ 4. One of the first steps to completing a functional assessment is:
(a) Describing the target behavior; assigning an operational definition
(b) Understanding the behavior from the perspective of the person who directly observes it and the problem it causes for other people
(c) Identifying the patterns of triggers to help figure out how a behavior is maintained
(d) Assessing the effectiveness of different approaches on the target behavior

_____ 5. Which of the following is the most suggestive indicator that a behavior pattern may be the result of a mental illness:
(a) The behavior is exhibited only at home
(b) The behavior occurs in all environments; it is not observed just in specific settings
(c) The behavior never occurs when the person's favorite direct support professional is supporting him/her
(d) The person appears to be able to start and stop the behavior at will

_____ 6. The bio-psycho-social model _____
(a) Does not require the review of existing data or background information to contribute to

the assessment process

(b) Recognizes that mental health is defined only by the relative absence of psychological distress

(c) Incorporates the effects of biomedical and psychological factors and how these influences interrelate

(d) Recognizes that the clinical interview can be completed by reviewing the documented history and reports compiled about the person

_____ 7. Which of the following statements is accurate?

(a) Medical problems in people with IDD are easily recognized

(b) Dental problems in people with IDD are easily recognized

(c) Rapid onset in a change in behavior patterns is likely because behavioral problems are directly associated with having the condition of IDD

(d) Causes of self-injurious behavior in people with IDD can be related to an underlying medical condition

_____ 8. True or false: In addition to the client's health history (medical, psychological, substance use), clinicians should obtain the health history of family members.

_____ 9. True or false: People with IDD experience the full range of psychiatric disorders as compared to the general population.

_____ 10. Medical conditions:

(a) Can be present when behavioral problems are exhibited

(b) Are often underdiagnosed

(c) Can be masked as behavioral problems

(d) All of the above

M
O
D
U
L
E

3

Supplemental Materials

Module III: Comprehensive Assessment Practices

Comprehensive assessment practices encompass a set of procedures that help guide the clinician to a better clinical understanding of the individual. There are a number of components to this rather complex task.

A bio-psycho-social model of assessment is essential in the assessment process.

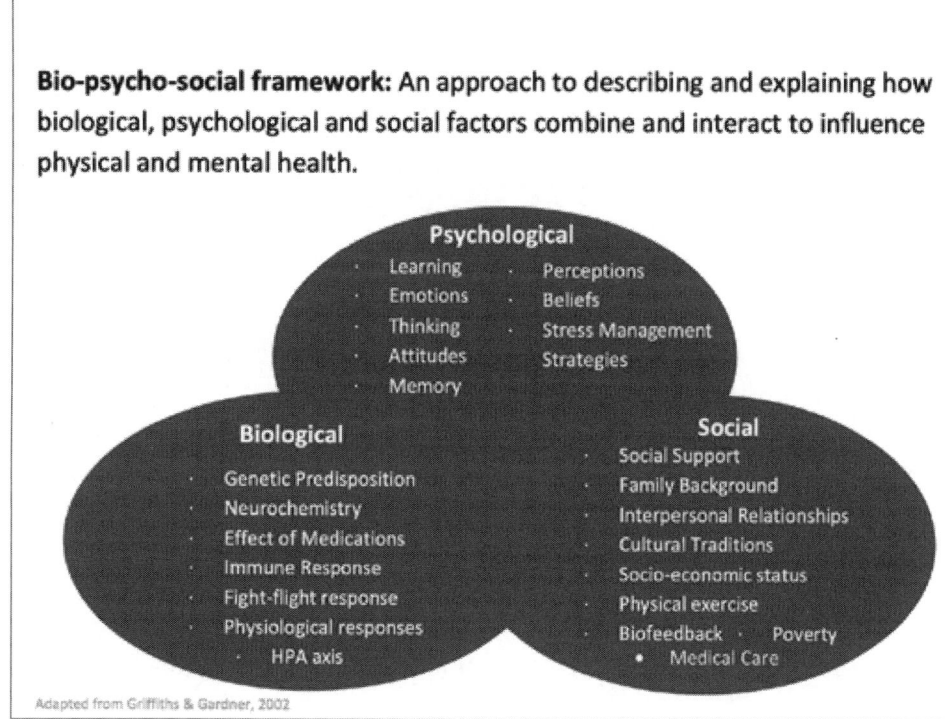

Bio-psycho-social framework: An approach to describing and explaining how biological, psychological and social factors combine and interact to influence physical and mental health.

Psychological
- Learning
- Emotions
- Thinking
- Attitudes
- Memory
- Perceptions
- Beliefs
- Stress Management Strategies

Biological
- Genetic Predisposition
- Neurochemistry
- Effect of Medications
- Immune Response
- Fight-flight response
- Physiological responses
- HPA axis

Social
- Social Support
- Family Background
- Interpersonal Relationships
- Cultural Traditions
- Socio-economic status
- Physical exercise
- Biofeedback · Poverty
- Medical Care

Adapted from Griffiths & Gardner, 2002

M
O
D
U
L
E

3

Exercises

Consider someone you know/support. Can you provide an example of how each of the factors of the bio-psycho-social model affects their mental health?

Biological

_____

_____

Psychological

_____

_____

Social

_____

_____

Medical problems and unmet health problems in people with IDD occur at a higher rate than in people in the general population. There is often a relationship between medical problems and problem behavior. Therefore, obtaining a recent medical assessment should be part of the overall assessment process.

Case Vignette

Mary is a 30-year-old female with a severe level of ID. She lives with her parents. Her mother expressed concern that Mary was pulling out her hair (trichotillomania). Upon a routine dental exam, the dentist observed an abscessed tooth and extracted it. Mary's mother reported that after the tooth was extracted, Mary ceased to pull out her hair.

Can you provide an example of the relationship between a medical issue and a problem behavior?

_____

_____

Stakeholder Reports

Obtaining reports from a variety of stakeholders is important to get a comprehensive assessment of what is observed and reported. These collateral contacts may include:

- Family members

- Health providers

- School personnel

- Mental health providers

- IDD providers

- Employers/vocational/day program staff

- Residential providers

- DSPs

- Other

Exercise

What is the value of obtaining information from Direct Support Professionals (DSPs)?

_____

_____

MODULE 3

Comprehensive Diagnostic Assessment

A comprehensive diagnostic assessment is complicated by numerous factors, including:

- Diagnostic overshadowing

- Problems with polypharmacy

- Communication deficits

- Atypical presentation of psychiatric disorders

- Limited life experiences

- Medical conditions

- Acquiescence

- Learned behavior

- Aggression and self-injurious behavior (SIB)

- Sensory impairment

- Behavioral overshadowing

- Medication masking

- Episodic presentation

- Division of services

- Lack of expertise

Exercise

Based on your experiences, give examples of diagnostic barriers. Can you explain how these barriers were overcome? If they were not overcome, what was the resulting impact?

Behavioral Status Review Reports

Conducting a mental health assessment with a person who has IDD is a very complex task. Documenting and communicating behavior changes is a team-based approach that should include family, caregivers, direct support professionals, clinicians and others with valuable information.

Recent Changes

In the chart below, the clinical team or care provider can indicate life changes that have occurred over the last six months. Any one of these items can contribute to or somehow be related to a behavioral health problem. This chart looks at changes in the environment that may affect behavior.

Name	Date
Person(s) completing form	
Recent moves or transitions	
Deaths of loved ones	
Loss of significant relationships	
Loss of pet	
Loss of key staff or teacher	
Change in health status	
Change in medication	
Evidence of other grief reaction	
Change or loss of employment	
Change or loss of program or service	
Change or loss of hobby or recreation	
Other remarkable changes	

M
O
D
U
L
E

3

Observable Behavior

This is another chart that can assist in the assessment process. In this chart, we are looking at areas that may be indicative, but not necessarily proof, of a mental health disorder.

The clinical team or care provider checks off whether the observable behavior is chronic, acute, episodic or non-applicable. Remember to document that which you can see.

When questioning regarding self-injury, the clinician must receive a detailed, precise description of the problem behavior (e.g., SIB — punching self with closed fist vs. slapping one's face). Clarity around exactly what the behavior looks like is vital for accurate assessment.

Name		Date				
Person(s) completing form						
Behavior (include concrete description)	C	A	E	NA	Additional comments/info	
Aggression						
Self-injury						
Appears anxious						
Excessive worrying						
Appears hypervigilant						
Engages in rituals/compulsions						
Steals						
Hoards items						
Impulsivity						
Verbal threats						
Physical threats						
Circle: increase or decrease in eating						
Circle: increase or decrease in sleeping						
Circle: increase or decrease in energy						
Circle: increase or decrease in social activity						
Circle: increase or decrease in hygiene						

Chronic: Person displays behavior on a daily basis, across settings
Acute: Behavior represents a dramatic change and occurs inconsistently
Episodic: Periods of disturbance and periods of normal functioning
N/A: Non-Applicable

MODULE 3

Quality-of-Life Issues

The assessment process should also include listing the positive attributes, desires and pleasurable activities of the individual. This can include not only activities enjoyed by the person, but also important relationships involved in the person's life. The chart below is not exhaustive but can provide some examples and opportunities for improvement.

Please explain more about the areas below that the person enjoys and that promote quality of life:

	Description	Satisfactory	Needs improvement
Family			
Friends			
Romance			
Living situation/home			
Leisure/hobbies			
Work/employment			
School			
Staff and support			
Diet and nutrition			
Exercise and wellness			
Mental health supports			
Privacy			
Finances			
Safety			
Worship and spirituality			
Neighborhood/community			
Other			
Other			

A valuable toolkit for working with someone with communication difficulties is available at http://iddtoolkit.vkcsites.org/general-issues/communicating-effectively/

MODULE 3

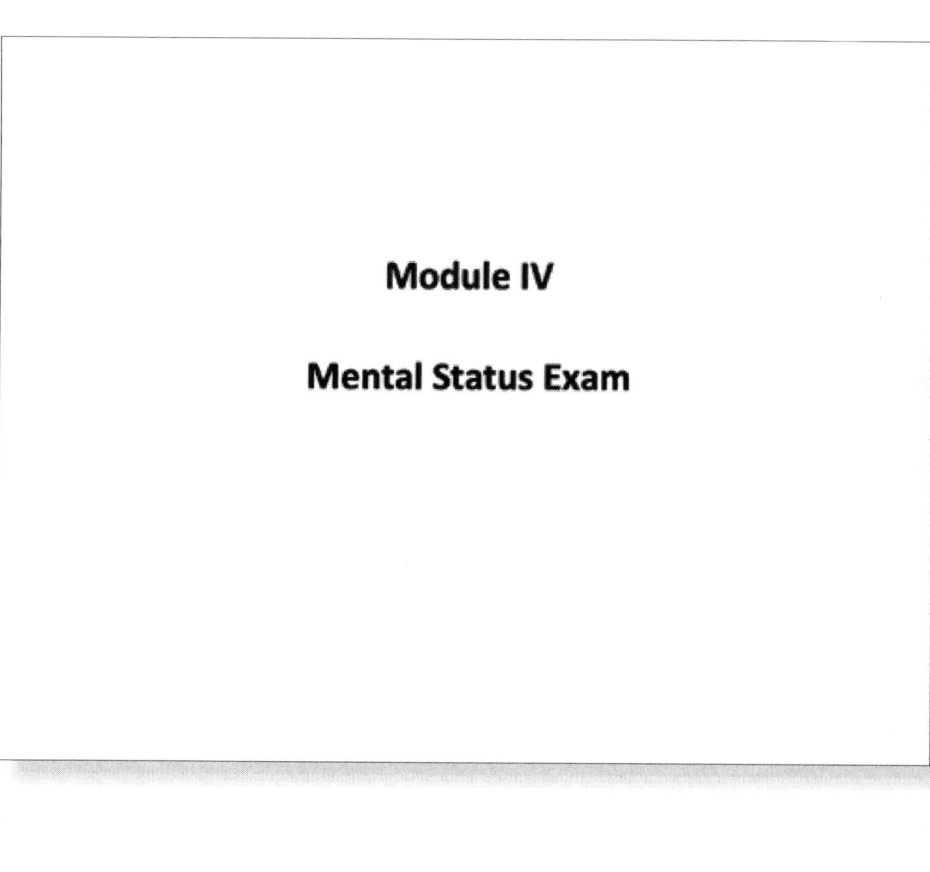

Module IV

Mental Status Exam

Pre-test

Module IV: Mental Status Exam

_____ 1.   True or false: The Mental Status Exam (MSE) is intended to be part of a comprehensive assessment of a person's overall condition at the time the exam is administered.

_____ 2.   The higher-level functions of the brain involved in gaining knowledge and comprehension are referred to as:
(a) Theory of mind
(b) Stream-of-consciousness thought
(c) Cognitive functions
(d) Functional analysis

_____ 3.   Which one is not a common challenge encountered when completing a proper diagnosis for a person who has an intellectual/developmental disability and a mental health problem?
(a) Intellectual distortion
(b) Baseline exaggeration
(c) Lack of independent identity
(d) Psycho-social masking

_____ 4.   True or false: When completing a Mental Status Exam (MSE), the clinician does not need to have an understanding of the person's baseline behavior since the MSE only provides a quick snapshot of the mental status at the time of the assessment.

_____ 5.   Assessment of mood and affect involves assessing and:
(a) Describing the predominant mood and its impact on others
(b) Describing how the person responds to intentional changes in affect of the clinician
(c) Describing the predominant mood of the person and the person's outward expression of internal emotions
(d) Describing the general atmosphere of the assessment environment to interpret the impact on the assessment process

_____ 6.   Fill in the blank: _____ can be a significant problem for making a good diagnosis as care providers may see only the escalation of the problem behavior rather than note it along with other symptoms of a psychiatric disorder.
(a) Effective field theory
(b) Hashimoto's disease
(c) Baseline exaggeration

(d) Paparazzi effect

_____ 7. True or false: People with IDD may have preexisting challenges with hyperactivity, challenges with gait, coordination and verbal communication that need to be understood by the clinician when conducting the MSE.

_____ 8. When assessing thought process and content as part of the MSE, which of the following is not a consideration?
(a) Obsessions
(b) Self-talk
(c) Telekinesis
(d) Phobias

_____ 9. When assessing cognitive function in a person who has an intellectual/developmental disability, a clinician would not consider:
(a) Attention and concentration
(b) Developmental level
(c) Memory
(d) Daily living skills

_____ 10. True or false: Judgment and insight cannot be assessed for a person with an intellectual/developmental disability.

M
O
D
U
L
E

4

Slide 1

Module IV

Mental Status Exam

Slide 2

This module includes information about best practices in mental health evaluation for persons with IDD with a focus on mental status examination (MSE).

Slide 3

Learning Objectives

- Summarize the importance of assessing the cognitive developmental level of the person with IDD as it pertains to Mental Status Examination.
- Describe the 11 domains and how they are pertinent to the assessment process.
- Describe how the developmental level of the person is related to the assessment process.

Slide 4

Definitions

Affect: The observable expression of emotion

Psychomotor activity: Movement or muscle activity related to mental processes

Thought process: Brain processing information to form concepts, make decisions, reason and problem-solve

Cognitive functions: The mental processes involved in gaining knowledge and comprehension—thinking, knowing, remembering, judging and problem-solving. These are higher-level functions of the brain and encompass language, imagination, perception and planning.

Judgment: Process by which people make decisions and form conclusions based on available information and material combined with thought and experience

Insight: Self-understanding—the awareness of own attitudes, feelings and behavior

Slide 5

Effects of IDD in Clinical Presentation

The interaction between IDD and MI is a result of four factors that reflect the profound bio-psycho-social effects of developmental disabilities:

1. Intellectual distortion

2. Psycho-social masking

3. Cognitive disintegration

4. Baseline exaggeration

Sovner, 1986

Slide 6

Four Nonspecific Factors Associated with IDD that Influence the Diagnostic Process

Factor 1: Intellectual Distortion

Definition: Refers to the developmental effects of IDD on the person's diminished ability to think abstractly and communicate intelligibly.

Clinical Impact: Inability for person to label their own experiences and report them.

Example: When asked if they "hear voices," the person might respond "yes" without fully comprehending the implication of the question.

Sovner, 1986

Slide 7

Four Nonspecific Factors Associated with IDD that Influence the Diagnostic Process

Factor 2: Psycho-social Masking

Definition: Impoverished social skills and life experiences can influence the content of psychiatric symptoms.

Clinical Impact: The person with IDD might present significant symptomatology that occurs within the developmental framework.

Example: A person with a moderate level of IDD might believe they can drive a car, and this can be a manifestation of grandiosity.

Sovner, 1986

Slide 8

Four Nonspecific Factors Associated with IDD that Influence the Diagnostic Process

Factor 3: Cognitive Disintegration

Definition: Stress-induced disruption of information processing— Tendency of person with IDD to become disorganized under stress.

Clinical Impact: Bizarre presentation and psychotic-like state may be misdiagnosed as schizophrenia.

Example: Vulnerability to high levels of stress and overload of cognitive functioning may lead to atypical clinical presentation.

Sovner, 1986

Slide 9

Four Nonspecific Factors Associated with IDD that Influence the Diagnostic Process

Factor 4: Baseline Exaggeration

Definition: Preexisting maladaptive behaviors that were not attributed to mental illness may increase in frequency and intensity with the onset of a psychiatric disorder.

Clinical Impact: Creates difficulty in establishing illness features, target symptoms and outcome measures.

Example: SIB (Self-Injurious Behavior) or aggression that occurred infrequently may suddenly increase in severity at onset of a psychiatric disorder.

Sovner, 1986

Slide 10

- The Mental Status Exam can only be administered by a regulated health or mental health professional such as a physician, nurse, psychologist or psychiatrist.

- A direct support professional can contribute to the process by being familiar with the components of the exam and the information they may need to assist the person to receive an accurate assessment.

Slide 11

A Mental Status Exam is a brief assessment intended to provide a snapshot of the mental status of the person at the time of the assessment.

Levitas, Hurley & Pary, 2001

Slide 12

- Systematic observation and recording about a person's thinking, emotions and behavior

- MSE for people with IDD needs to be modified

- Useful way to organize and standardize the data of patient observation

- MSE is a snapshot of the mental status at the time of the assessment. The MSE can be used as a tool to note change in the status from one point in time to another.

- MSE is a diagnostic measurement. Data from care providers and patient history can be helpful.

Levitas, Hurley & Pary, 2001

M
O
D
U
L
E

4

Slide 13

I.   General appearance and behavior

II. Mood and affect

III. Psychomotor activity and speech

IV. Thought process and content

V.   Cognitive function

VI. Judgment and insight

Levitas, Hurley & Pary, 2001

Slide 14

Case Study

As we work through each section of the mental status exam, we will consider the case of Ms. Thao. This is the examiner's first appointment with Ms. Thao. The results of the assessment will serve as the baseline for noting change in Ms. Thao's mental health.

Levitas, Hurley & Pary, 2001

Slide 15

I.   **General appearance and behavior**

- Assess person's attentiveness and effective participation in interview
- Note person's attitude toward examiner
- Assess posture and general motor activity
- Note facial expression
- Note personal hygiene and grooming
- Assess weight status

Note: All of the above are based on the cognitive developmental level of the individual with IDD.

Levitas, Hurley & Pary, 2001

M
O
D
U
L
E

4

Slide 16

I. General appearance and behavior (cont.)

- The clinician may need to rely on collateral information about the person's baseline appearance and behavior.

- Baseline for a person with IDD may be very different from the neurotypical person. For example, in a person with ASD, body posturing, self-hugging and finger-flicking may be the typical baseline behavior for a person on the spectrum.

Note: All of the above are based on the cognitive developmental level of the individual with IDD.

Levitas, Hurley & Pary, 2001

Slide 17

I. General appearance and behavior — Ms. Thao

- Wearing loose-fitting T-shirt and dress customary for her ethnicity

- The examiner has no further ability to determine gender

- Eye contact averted for first 10 minutes of the exam

- Following first 10 minutes, Ms. Thao was attentive and engaged, speaking freely and unguarded.

- Ms. Thao was neatly groomed with unremarkable hygiene.

Levitas, Hurley & Pary, 2001

Slide 18

- Ms. Thao appears to be underweight.

- She displayed a high level of motor activity. Her facial expression appeared worried.

- She fidgeted and squirmed frequently.

- Ms. Thao did smile and laugh periodically.

- Ms. Thao's care providers reported her appearance and behavior as typical.

- Ms. Thao's posture and appearance of muscle tone were unremarkable.

- Ms. Thao wrung her hands and adjusted her clothing repeatedly

Levitas, Hurley & Pary, 2001

Slide 19

Exercise

I. General Appearance

- Body build
- Appropriate clothing
- Clean, neat, tidy
- Hygiene and grooming
- Odor
- Facial expression
- Eye contact
- Other things that are noteworthy

Levitas, Hurley & Pary, 2001

Slide 20

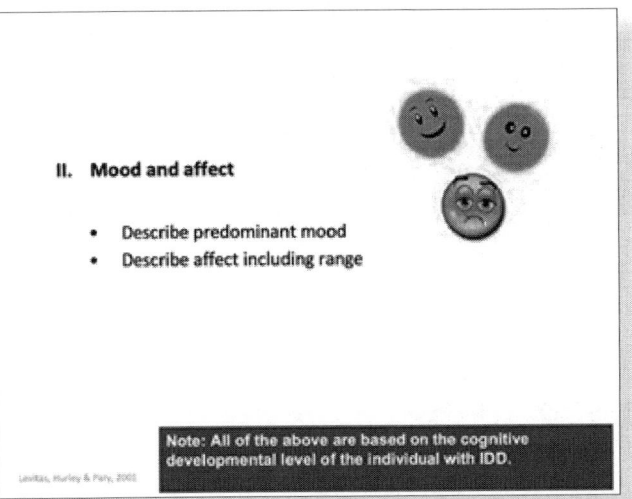

II. Mood and affect

- Describe predominant mood
- Describe affect including range

Note: All of the above are based on the cognitive developmental level of the individual with IDD.

Levitas, Hurley & Pary, 2001

Slide 21

II. Mood and affect (cont.)

- Mood is the prevailing emotional state. Affect is the expression of emotions.
- An examiner can draw faces to help the client identify feeling state.
    - Ask person to point to face to show how he/she is feeling today.

Happy Sad Mad Fearful Neutral

Note: All of the above are based on the cognitive developmental level of the individual with IDD.

Levitas, Hurley & Pary, 2001

Slide 22

II. Mood and affect — Ms. Thao

- Ms. Thao exhibited high levels of anxiety throughout the visit. This was her predominant emotional state.

- Her range of emotion displayed included mild euphoria when describing family, pets and gardening.

- Ms. Thao appeared to be quite worried about numerous topics, including street gangs, burglary and graffiti.

Levitas, Hurley & Pary, 2001

Slide 23

Exercise

II. Mood and affect

- Appropriateness of affect/appropriate or inappropriate to situation. Congruous/incongruous
- Range of affect
- Stability of affect
- Attitude during encounter
- Specific mood or feelings, observed or reported
- Anxiety level rate

Levitas, Hurley & Pary, 2001

Slide 24

III. Psychomotor activity and speech

- Assess psychomotor activity and notes
    - Rate of psychomotor activity (e.g., agitated, slowed)
    - Presence of abnormal movements (grimacing, mannerisms, stereotype)
- Assess speech and note amount, volume, rate, organization of speech

Note: All of the above are based on the cognitive developmental level of the individual with IDD.

Levitas, Hurley & Pary, 2001

Slide 25

III. Psychomotor activity and speech (cont.)

- Examiner will need other collateral data in understanding the typical psychomotor activity and speech organization for the person.
    - For example, people who have Fragile X often have difficulty with gross motor coordination, which may lead to assessment as abnormal movements in absence of information about the effect of the syndrome.

Note: All of the above are based on the cognitive developmental level of the individual with IDD.

Levitas, Hurley & Pary, 2001

Slide 26

III. Psychomotor activity and speech — Ms. Thao

- Ms. Thao exhibited a high level of motor activity, frequently fidgeting, wringing her hands and adjusting clothing.

- No abnormal movements were observed.

- Ms. Thao's speech was easily understandable.

- Ms. Thao spoke rapidly and in an animated manner no matter what the topic was.

- Ms. Thao made numerous repetitive statements about criminal activity.

- Much of the discussion with Ms. Thao focused on past worrisome events, including a history of cutting.

Levitas, Hurley & Pary, 2001

Slide 27

Exercise

III. Psychomotor behavior

- Gait
- Handshake
- Abnormal movements
- Posture
- Rate of movements
- Coordination

Levitas, Hurley & Pary, 2001

Slide 28

IV. Thought process and content

- Assess thought abnormalities
- Evaluate the content of thought
- Note presence of delusions/hallucinations (if so, note type of hallucinations)

Note: All of the above are based on the cognitive developmental level of the individual with IDD.

Levitas, Hurley & Pary, 2001

Slide 29

IV. Thought process and content (cont.)

- Clinical challenge in identifying abnormal thoughts and perceptions related to mental illness, compared to behaviors associated with the cognitive/developmental level of the individual
- Similarities between behaviors normal in young children without IDD and adults with IDD (i.e., self-talk, imaginary friends and rich fantasy life)

Note: All of the above are based on the cognitive developmental level of the individual with IDD.

Levitas, Hurley & Pary, 2001

Slide 30

IV. Thought process and content — Ms. Thao

- Ms. Thao's thought process appeared to be clear, though jumping from one source of worry to another and frequently revisiting past topics.
- Ms. Thao displayed directed attention to the interviewer.
- There was no evidence of delusional thinking nor significant fantasy life.
- Ms. Thao had difficulty staying focused on a single topic, though she could be redirected back to a topic of conversation.

Levitas, Hurley & Pary, 2001

MODULE 4

Slide 31

Exercise

IV. Thought process and content
- Clarity
- Relevance/logic
- Flow
- Rapidly shifting ideas/thoughts
- Perseveration
- Pressure of speech
- Thoughts/content consistent with reality

Levitas, Hurley & Pary, 2001

Slide 32

V. Cognitive function

- Assess orientations to time, place and persons
- Evaluate attention and concentration
- Assess memory
- Assess intellectual functioning

Note: All of the above are based on the cognitive
developmental level of the individual with IDD.

Levitas, Hurley & Pary, 2001

Slide 33

V. Cognitive function (cont.)
- Detailed information and chronology of events need to be considered relative to the person's developmental age. For example, they may remember the names of their siblings and know which are older and younger but may not be able to remember the exact age of each sibling.
- The examiner will need to assess intellectual functioning based on estimating the person's level of functioning.

Note: All of the above are based on the cognitive
developmental level of the individual with IDD.

Levitas, Hurley & Pary, 2001

Slide 34

V. Cognitive function — Ms. Thao

- Ms. Thao understood time, place and persons and also understood the nature of the meeting.

- Ms. Thao successfully gave the observer a tour of her home and understood the roles of her family and people paid to provide her with support.

- Ms. Thao had displayed difficulty with crude recall of facts, although she clearly remembered criminal activity around her neighborhood and described gang signs.

Levitas, Hurley & Pary, 2001

Slide 35

Exercise

V. Cognitive function

- Attention and concentration
- Memory
- Abstraction concrete thinking
- Orientation

Levitas, Hurley & Pary, 2001

Slide 36

VI. Judgment and insight

- Assess judgment in general
- Evaluate insight in situation and illness

Note: All of the above are based on the cognitive developmental level of the individual with IDD.

Levitas, Hurley & Pary, 2001

M
O
D
U
L
E

4

Slide 37

VI. Judgment and insight — Ms. Thao

- The examiner observed Ms. Thao had insight into her anxiety to the degree that she was aware she worried more than her family members, but felt her additional worry was smart and reasonable.

- Ms. Thao was unable to offer insight into the nature of her worry.

Levitas, Hurley & Pary, 2001

Slide 38

Exercise

VI. Judgment and insight

- Impulsive behavior
- Insight into illness
- Examples

Levitas, Hurley & Pary, 2001

M
O
D
U
L
E

4

Post-test

Module IV: Mental Status Exam

_____ 1.   True or false: The Mental Status Exam (MSE) is intended to be part of a comprehensive assessment of a person's overall condition at the time the exam is administered.

_____ 2.   The higher-level functions of the brain involved in gaining knowledge and comprehension are referred to as:
(a) Theory of mind
(b) Stream-of-consciousness thought
(c) Cognitive functions
(d) Functional analysis

_____ 3.   Which one is not a common challenge encountered when completing a proper diagnosis for a person who has an intellectual/developmental disability and a mental health problem?
(a) Intellectual distortion
(b) Baseline exaggeration
(c) Lack of independent identity
(d) Psycho-social masking

_____ 4.   True or false: When completing a Mental Status Exam (MSE), the clinician does not need to have an understanding of the person's baseline behavior since the MSE only provides a quick snapshot of the mental status at the time of the assessment.

_____ 5.   Assessment of mood and affect involves assessing and:
(a) Describing the predominant mood and its impact on others
(b) Describing how the person responds to intentional changes in affect of the clinician
(c) Describing the predominant mood of the person and the person's outward expression of internal emotions
(d) Describing the general atmosphere of the assessment environment to interpret the impact on the assessment process

_____ 6.   Fill in the blank: _____ can be a significant problem for making a good diagnosis as care providers may see only the escalation of the problem behavior rather than note it along with other symptoms of a psychiatric disorder.
(a) Effective field theory
(b) Hashimoto's disease
(c) Baseline exaggeration
(d) Paparazzi effect

MODULE 4

_____ 7. True or false: People with IDD may have preexisting challenges with hyperactivity, challenges with gait, coordination and verbal communication that need to be understood by the clinician when conducting the MSE.

_____ 8. When assessing thought process and content as part of the MSE, which of the following is not a consideration?
(a) Obsessions
(b) Self-talk
(c) Telekinesis
(d) Phobias

_____ 9. When assessing cognitive function in a person who has an intellectual/developmental disability, a clinician would not consider:
(a) Attention and concentration
(b) Developmental level
(c) Memory
(d) Daily living skills

_____ 10. True or false: Judgment and insight cannot be assessed for a person with an intellectual/developmental disability.

MODULE 4

Supplemental Materials

Module IV: Mental Status Exam

Definitions

We give you a number of definitions for terms used in this module that describe how we sum up a person's mental state. Review them, and then imagine you run into a friend you haven't seen in a while. You have heard from other friends that this person has been having a rough time. Do these terms include all the things you would consider when you thought about how your friend was doing? Why or why not?

_____

_____

IDD and Clinical Presentation

These four considerations are discussed a lot in this module. They all influence how mental health might appear in a person with disabilities. Please think of one example of each of these four topic areas as shown by people you have supported:

1. Intellectual distortion

   _____

   _____

2. Psycho-social masking

   _____

   _____

3. Cognitive disintegration

   _____

   _____

4. Baseline exaggeration

_____

_____

The Mental Status Exam

Part 1: Try to practice doing a few quick summaries of Mental Status as described in this module. Observe three people whom you support, and write down what you observe for each of the six sections of an MSE.

Part 2: Mental Status Exams also ask questions to determine if a person can answer simple questions about what is going on in the world. Common questions might include who the president is, what cars the person has driven or recent events. These questions might be difficult for people with disabilities. For each of the people you think about in this exercise, write down three questions you could ask the person to see if they were aware of things happening in their life.

Person 1

1. General Appearance and Behavior

_____

_____

2. Mood and Affect

_____

_____

3. Psychomotor Activity and Speech

_____

_____

4. Thought Process and Content

_____

_____

5. Cognitive Function

_____

_____

6. Judgment and Insight

_____

_____

Question 1:

_____

_____

Question 2:

_____

_____

Question 3:

_____

_____

M
O
D
U
L
E

4

Person 2

1. General Appearance and Behavior

_____

_____

2. Mood and Affect

_____

_____

3. Psychomotor Activity and Speech

_____

_____

4. Thought Process and Content

_____

_____

5. Cognitive Function

_____

_____

6. Judgment and Insight

_____

_____

Question 1:

_____

Question 2:

Question 3:

Person 3

1. General Appearance and Behavior

2. Mood and Affect

3. Psychomotor Activity and Speech

4. Thought Process and Content

5. Cognitive Function

_____

_____

6. Judgment and Insight

_____

_____

Question 1:

_____

_____

Question 2:

_____

_____

Question 3:

_____

_____

Now, remember the situation we gave you when you ran into an old friend in a store? Look at the different areas considered in a Mental Status Exam. Once again, are these topic areas the ones you would consider when thinking about how your friend was doing? Why or why not? Please explain your thinking.

Module V

Overview of the Diagnostic Manual for Persons with Intellectual Disability (DM-ID-2)

Pre-test

Module V: Overview of the Diagnostic Manual for Persons with Intellectual Disability (DM-ID-2)

_____ 1.   The DM-ID-2 was developed in part because of which of the following:
(a) The DSM-5 relies on self-reporting of signs and symptoms, which is difficult to ascertain in individuals with IDD
(b) Diagnostic categories are different for people with IDD
(c) The DSM-5 is a reliable tool for diagnosing individuals with IDD
(d) The greater the IDD, the more reliable was the DSM-5

_____ 2.   The DM-ID-2 diagnostic system _____
(a) Focuses on comparing the DSM and the International Classification System (ICD)
(b) Focuses on the International Classification System (ICD)
(c) Compares the DSM-5 and the DM-ID-2 diagnostic criteria
(d) All of the above

_____ 3.   Psychiatric diagnosis tends to _____
(a) Vary greatly from person to person
(b) Require biological markers
(c) Differ only by age
(d) Not apply to children

_____ 4.   Which of the following is *not* something clinicians should do when speaking to an individual with IDD:
(a) Speak in a monotone voice
(b) Ask one simple question at a time
(c) Wait for the answers before proceeding
(d) Use visuals

_____ 5.   True or false: In the assessment process, information on individuals with IDD should be provided only by clinicians and staff.

_____ 6.   True or false: Behavioral phenotype denotes a set of behaviors that are genetically determined and are associated with a particular genetic disorder.

_____ 7.   True or false: The DM-ID-2 is an acronym to describe people with IDD.

**M
O
D
U
L
E

5**

_____ 8. Which of the following is not an adaptation used in the DM-ID-2?
(a) Modification of symptom duration
(b) Changes in symptom count
(c) Addition on symptom equivalents
(d) Use of medications

_____ 9. A _____ perspective is emphasized throughout the DM-ID-2 to assist the clinician in recognizing psychiatric disorders.
(a) Developmental
(b) Depressive
(c) Reactive
(d) Childhood

_____ 10. An accurate DM-ID-2 diagnosis can lead to all of the following except:
(a) Effective treatment
(b) An increase in the level of IQ
(c) Better quality of life
(d) Improved outcomes

MODULE 5

MODULE 5

Slide 1

Module V

Overview of the Diagnostic Manual for Persons with Intellectual Disability (DM-ID-2)

Slide 2

This module contains information about the DM-ID-2 and how it can assist in the diagnostic process with persons with IDD.

Slide 3

Learning Objectives

- Describe the impact of the DM-ID-2 on the diagnostic process as compared to the DSM-5.
- Articulate the types of adaptations made in the DM-ID-2.
- Describe several adaptations as they compare to the DSM-5 in diagnostic subsets.

Slide 4

Limitations of DSM-5 System

- Diagnostic overshadowing (Reiss et al., 1982)
- Applicability of established diagnostic systems is increasingly suspect as the severity of ID increases (Rush, 2000)
- DSM-5 system relies on self report of signs and symptoms

Slide 5

DM-ID-2: Two Manuals

Diagnostic Manual—Intellectual Disability: A Textbook of Diagnosis of Mental Disorders in Persons with Intellectual Disability-2

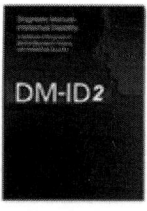

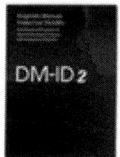

Diagnostic Manual—Intellectual Disability: A Clinical Guide for Diagnosis of Mental Disorders in Persons with Intellectual Disability-2

Slide 6

Overview of the DM-ID-2

- An adaptation to the DSM-5
- Designed to facilitate a more accurate psychiatric diagnosis
- Based on expert consensus model
- Covers all major diagnostic categories as defined in DSM-5

DM-ID-2

Slide 7

Overview of the DM-ID-2

- Provides information to help with diagnostic process
- Addresses pathoplastic effect of ID on psychopathology (disorder of expression)
- Designed with a developmental perspective to help clinicians recognize symptom profiles in adults and children with ID

DM-ID-2

Slide 8

Overview of the DM-ID-2

- Provides state-of-the-art information about mental disorders in persons with ID
- Provides adaptations of criteria, where appropriate

DM-ID-2

Slide 9

Two Special Added-Value Chapters

- Assessment and Diagnostic Procedures
- Behavioral Phenotype of Genetic Disorders

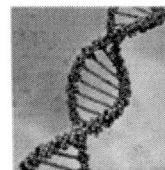

DM-ID-2

Slide 10

Assessment and Diagnostic Procedures

Special Consideration: Language That Is Understandable

- Use simple language
- Create short sentences
- Check back with person for understanding
- Use examples

DM-ID-2

Slide 11

Assessment and Diagnostic Procedures: Chapter 2

Assessment of Medical Conditions

- Constipation → distress
- Hypothyroidism → depressive symptoms
- Hyperthyroidism → manic episode
- Diabetes → behavioral side effects

DM-ID-2

Slide 12

Behavioral Phenotype of Genetic Disorders: Chapter 3

Angelman syndrome	Prader-Willi syndrome
Cri-du-Chat (5p-) syndrome	Rubinstein-Taybi syndrome
Down syndrome	Smith-Magenis syndrome
Fetal alcohol syndrome	Tuberous sclerosis complex
Fragile X syndrome	Velocardiofacial syndrome
Phenylketonuria	Williams syndrome

DM-ID-2

MODULE 5

Slide 13

Behavioral Phenotype of Genetic Disorders: Chapter 3

Down syndrome

Phenotype	Small head, mouth; upward slant to eyes; epicanthal folds; broad neck; hypothyroidism; hearing loss; visual impairments; cardiac problems; gastrointestinal; orthopedic and skin disorders; obesity	
Behavioral Phenotype	Childhood	Oppositional and defiant; attention-deficit/hyperactivity disorder (ADHD); social, charming personality "stereotype"
	Adulthood	Depressive disorders; obsessive-compulsive disorder; other anxiety disorders; dementia of the Alzheimer's type; mental disorders associated with hypothyroidism

DM-ID-2

Slide 14

DM-ID-2
Diagnostic Chapter Structure

- Review of diagnostic criteria
  - General description of the disorder
  - Summary of DSM-5 criteria
- Issues related to diagnosis in people with ID
- Review of literature/research

DM-ID-2

Slide 15

Application of Diagnostic Criteria to People with ID

- General considerations
- Adults with mild to moderate ID
- Adults with severe or profound ID
- Children and adolescents with ID

DM-ID-2

Slide 16

Etiology and Pathogenesis

• Risk factors
- Biological factors
- Psychological factors
- Genetic syndromes

DM-ID-2

Slide 17

Diagnostic Criteria

DSM-5 Criteria	Criteria Mild-Moderate ID	Criteria Severe-Profound ID

DM-ID-2

Slide 18

Adaptation of the DSM-5 Criteria

1. Addition of symptom equivalents
2. Does not apply
3. Changes in symptom count
4. Modification of symptom duration
5. Modification of age requirements
6. Addition of explanatory notes

DM-ID-2

Slide 19

Adaptation of DSM-5 Criteria
Addition of Symptom Equivalent
Social Anxiety Disorder

DSM-5 Criteria	Adapted Criteria for Mild and Moderate ID	Adapted Criteria for Severe and Profound ID
A. Marked fear or anxiety about one or more social situations in which the individual is exposed to possible scrutiny by others. Examples include social interactions (e.g., eating or drinking) and performing in front of others.	No adaptation for mild ID. For moderate ID, anxiety occurs in peer settings.	Fear can be observed rather than subjectively described or expressed by crying, tantrums, freezing, clinging, shrinking, failure to speak in social situations.

Slide 20

Adaptation of DSM-5 Criteria
Symptoms that do not apply
Delusional Disorder

DSM-5 Criteria	Adapted Criteria for Mild & Moderate ID	Adapted Criteria for Severe & Profound ID
A. The presence of one (or more) delusions with a duration of one month or longer.	No adaptation	Does not apply
D. If manic or major depressive episodes have occurred, these have been brief relative to the duration of the delusional periods.	No adaptation	Does not apply

Slide 21

Adaptation of DSM-5 Criteria
Change in Count and Symptom Equivalent
Major Depressive Disorder

DSM-5 Criteria	Adapted Criteria for Mild to Profound IDD
A. Five or more of the following symptoms have been present during the same two-week period and represent a change from previous functioning. At least one of the symptoms is either (1) depressed mood or (2) loss of interest or pleasure.	A. Four or more symptoms have been present during the same two-week period and represent a change from previous functioning. At least one of the symptoms is either (1) depressed mood or (2) loss of interest or pleasure or (3) irritable mood.

Slide 22

Adaptation of DSM-5 Criteria
Modification Symptom Duration
Adjustment Disorder

DSM-5 Criteria	Applying Criteria for Mild to moderate ID	Applying Criteria for severe/profound ID
E. Once the stressor or its consequences have terminated, the symptoms do not persist for six (6) additional months.	An adjustment disorder must resolve within six months of the termination of the stressor (or its consequences). However, the symptoms may persist for a longer period (i.e., longer than six months) if they occur in response to a chronic stressor.	An adjustment disorder must resolve within six months of the termination of the stressor (or its consequences). However, the symptoms may persist for a longer period (i.e., longer than six months) if they occur in response to a chronic stressor.

DM-ID-2

Slide 23

Adaptation of DSM-5 Criteria
Modification of Age Requirement
Antisocial Personality Disorder

DSM-5 Criteria	Adapted Criteria for Individuals with ID
A. There is a pervasive pattern of disregard for and violation of the rights of others occurring since age 15 years, as indicated by three (or more) of the following:	A. There is a pervasive pattern of disregard for and violation of the rights of others occurring since age 18 years, as indicated by three (or more) of the following:
B. The individual is at least age 18 years.	B. The individual is at least age 21 years.
C. There is evidence of conduct disorder with the onset before age 15 years.	C. There is evidence of conduct disorder with onset before age 18 years.

DM-ID-2

Slide 24

Adaptation of Criteria
Addition of Explanatory Note
Manic Episode

DSM-IV-TR Criteria	Applying Criteria for Mild to Profound IDD
A. A distinct period of abnormally persistently elevated, expansive or irritable mood, lasting at least one week (or any duration if hospitalization is necessary).	A. No adaptation. Note: Observers may report that the individual with IDD has loud, inappropriate laughing or singing; is excessively giddy or silly; is intrusive, getting into other's space; and smiles excessively and in ways that are not appropriate to the social context. Elated mood may be alternating with irritable mood.

DSM-ID-2007

Slide 25

DM-ID-2 Improves Lives
Accurate Diagnosis
Effective Treatment
Improved Outcomes
Better Quality of Life

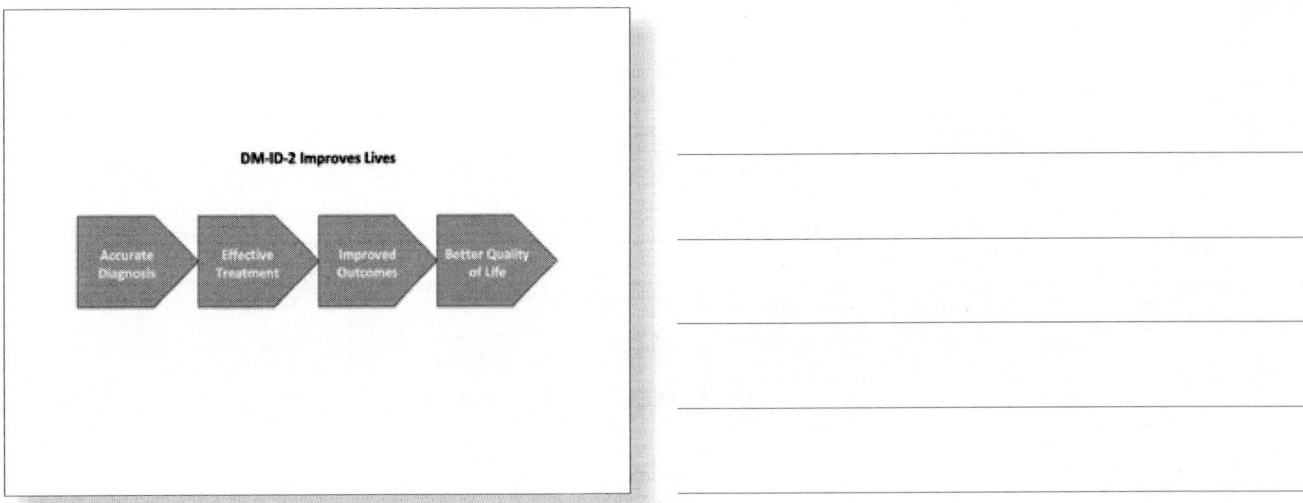

Post-test

Module V: Overview of the Diagnostic Manual for Persons with Intellectual Disability (DM-ID-2)

_____ 1. The DM-ID-2 was developed in part because of which of the following:
(a) The DSM-5 relies on self-reporting of signs and symptoms, which is difficult to ascertain in individuals with IDD
(b) Diagnostic categories are different for people with IDD
(c) The DSM-5 is a reliable tool for diagnosing individuals with IDD
(d) The greater the IDD, the more reliable was the DSM-5

_____ 2. The DM-ID-2 diagnostic system _____
(a) Focuses on comparing the DSM and the International Classification System (ICD)
(b) Focuses on the International Classification System (ICD)
(c) Compares the DSM-5 and the DM-ID-2 diagnostic criteria
(d) All of the above

_____ 3. Psychiatric diagnosis tends to _____
(a) Vary greatly from person to person
(b) Require biological markers
(c) Differ only by age
(d) Not apply to children

_____ 4. Which of the following is _not_ something clinicians should do when speaking to an individual with IDD:
(a) Speak in a monotone voice
(b) Ask one simple question at a time
(c) Wait for the answers before proceeding
(d) Use visuals

_____ 5. True or false: In the assessment process, information on individuals with IDD should be provided only by clinicians and staff.

_____ 6. True or false: Behavioral phenotype denotes a set of behaviors that are genetically determined and are associated with a particular genetic disorder.

_____ 7. True or false: The DM-ID-2 is an acronym to describe people with IDD.

M
O
D
U
L
E

5

_____ 8. Which of the following is not an adaptation used in the DM-ID-2?
(a) Modification of symptom duration
(b) Changes in symptom count
(c) Addition on symptom equivalents
(d) Use of medications

_____ 9. A _____ perspective is emphasized throughout the DM-ID-2 to assist the clinician in recognizing psychiatric disorders.
(a) Developmental
(b) Depressive
(c) Reactive
(d) Childhood

_____ 10. An accurate DM-ID-2 diagnosis can lead to all of the following except:
(a) Effective treatment
(b) An increase in the level of IQ
(c) Better quality of life
(d) Improved outcomes

M O D U L E 5

Supplemental Materials

Module V: Overview of the Diagnostic Manual for Persons with Intellectual Disability (DM-ID-2)

The comprehensive assessment and diagnostic practices entail gathering past and current information about the individual.

Exercise

List the types of data you would gather if you suspected a person is experiencing mental health symptoms.

The DM-ID-2 encompasses six types of modifications of the DSM criteria. These modifications are:

1. Addition of symptom equivalent
    Observed reports that are equivalent to self-reports

2. Criteria that do not apply or omissions of symptoms
    Criteria subsets that do not apply for people with severe/profound ID

3. Change in symptom count
    Indicated by frequency of symptoms that are required to meet diagnostic criteria.

4. Modification of symptom duration
    The length of time a symptom must be present in order to meet diagnostic criteria.

5. Modification of age
    Change in age in consideration of a developmental perspective

6. Addition of explanatory notes
    Intended to communicate a criterion without official modification of the criteria

M
O
D
U
L
E

5

Exercise

1. Can you identify a DM-ID-2 diagnosis in which one or more of these modifications apply? If so, explain.

   _____

   _____

2. Can you give an example of a symptom equivalent (observed reports that are equivalent to self-reports)?

   _____

   _____

3. Please explain why an accurate DM-ID-2 diagnosis is important for a positive clinical outcome for a person with IDD.

   _____

   _____

M
O
D
U
L
E

5

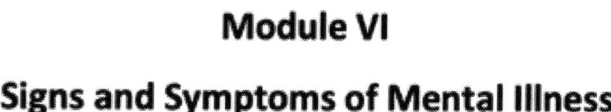

Module VI

Signs and Symptoms of Mental Illness

Pre-test

Module VI: Signs and Symptoms of Mental Illness

_____ 1.   What is the difference between anxiety people commonly feel in everyday life and having an anxiety disorder?
(a) Whether people see a therapist
(b) There is no difference
(c) Whether the anxiety interferes with quality of life
(d) If the person takes medication

_____ 2.   Which factor(s) can complicate diagnosis of mental health disorders in people with IDD?
(a) People with IDD may have narrow communication that can limit their ability to describe their symptoms
(b) People with IDD may experience symptoms of mental health disorders differently
(c) The symptoms a person is experiencing may be connected to a known IDD diagnosis, when there may actually be another condition
(d) All of the above

_____ 3.   True or false: Depression is not diagnosed as quickly for people with IDD as for the general population as onset tends to be more insidious and changes in baseline are not as apparent.

_____ 4.   _____ refers to the process of attributing all an individual's symptoms to a known condition.
(a) Assessment
(b) Diagnostic overshadowing
(c) Polypharmacy
(d) Screening

_____ 5.   True or false: A person with bipolar disorder will show cycling moods (periods of mania and periods of depression) over the course of days or hours.

_____ 6.   This disorder involves excessive anxiety or worry occurring more days than not for at least six months, about a number of events or activities:
(a) Phobia
(b) Generalized anxiety disorder
(c) Panic disorder
(d) Obsessive-compulsive disorder

M
O
D
U
L
E

6

_____ 7. _____ cause difficulty perceiving and relating to situations and people, including oneself.
(a) Personality disorders
(b) Mood disorders
(c) Phobias
(d) Compulsions

_____ 8. Psychosis may present in someone with IDD with which of the following symptoms?
(a) Delusions
(b) Hallucinations
(c) Disorganized speech
(d) All of the above

_____ 9. Which is an example of a wellness strategy to help manage anxiety?
(a) Avoiding work when feeling nervous
(b) Skipping a party where you don't know many people
(c) Staying awake all night and worrying about a test the next day
(d) Attending weekly yoga classes with a friend

_____ 10. Which is the greatest indicator that behaviors may indicate an underlying mental health condition?
(a) The behavior never occurs when the person is at work
(b) The behavior occurs less frequently if the person eats breakfast
(c) The behavior occurs in all environments/across settings
(d) The behavior is only observed at home

MODULE 6

Slide 1

Module VI

Signs and Symptoms of Mental Illness

Slide 2

This module includes information regarding signs and symptoms of depressive disorders, bipolar disorder, anxiety disorders, personality disorders and psychosis.

The module highlights the importance of observation of presentation of behavioral equivalents in people with IDD.

Slide 3

Learning Objectives

- Identify signs and symptoms of common mental health disorders
- Recognize presentation of behavioral equivalents mental health diagnoses in people with ID
- Recognize the importance of observation in the assessment process

M
O
D
U
L
E

6

Slide 4

Overview of the
Diagnostic Manual—Intellectual Disability, DM-ID-2

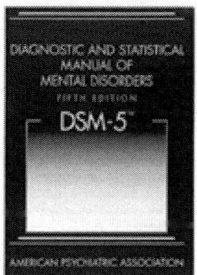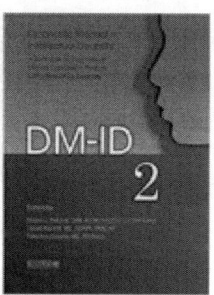

Slide 5

Diagnostic Challenges

- Communication
- Diagnostic overshadowing
- Acquiescence
- Appearing withdrawn
- Medications
- Behavioral
- Multiple diagnoses

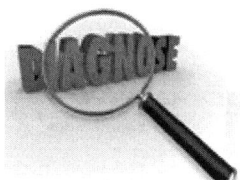

Slide 6

DEPRESSION

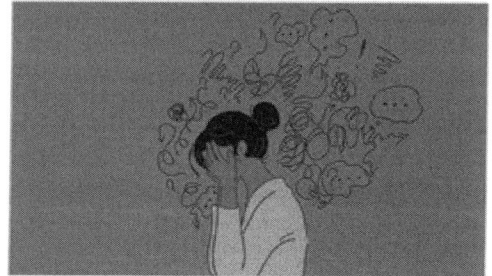

Slide 7

Depression

- Depression is characterized by low mood, accompanied by slowing of thinking and difficulty concentrating and sustaining energy.
- Can significantly disrupt school, work, family relationships, social life, hobbies.
- A loss of interest in pleasurable activities can be observed, i.e., the person no longer attending the activities from which he/she derived pleasure.
- Other symptoms include: Feelings of hopelessness or pessimism, appetite and/or weight changes and thoughts of death or suicide; suicide attempts.

Slide 8

Depression

Presentation in Someone with IDD
- Frequent unexplained crying
- Decrease in laughter and smiling
- General irritability and subsequent aggression or self-injury
- Sad facial expression
- No longer participates in favorite activities
- Reinforcers no longer valued
- Increased time spent alone
- Refusals of most work/social activities

DM-ID-2

Slide 9

Depression

Presentation in Someone with IDD
- Measured weight changes
- Increased refusals to come to table to eat
- Unusually disruptive at meal times
- Constant food-seeking behaviors
- Disruptive at bedtime
- Repeatedly gets up at night
- Difficulty falling asleep
- No longer gets up for work/activities
- Early-morning awakening
- Over 12 hours of sleep per day
- Naps frequently

DM-ID-2

MODULE 6

Slide 10

Depression

Presentation in Someone with IDD

- Sits for extended periods
- Moves slowly
- Takes longer than usual to complete activities
- Restless, fidgety, pacing
- Increased disruptive behavior

DM-ID-2

Slide 11

Depression

Presentation in Someone with IDD

- Needs frequent breaks to complete simple activity
- Slumped/tired body posture
- Does not complete tasks with multiple steps
- Statements like "I'm dumb," etc.
- Seeming to seek punishment
- Social isolation

DM-ID-2

Slide 12

Depression

Presentation in Someone with IDD

- Decreased work output
- Does not stay with tasks
- Decrease in IQ upon retesting
- Preoccupation with family member's death
- Talking about committing or attempting suicide
- Fascination with violent movies/television shows

DM-ID-2

Slide 13

Depression

Treatment Strategies

- Psychotherapy (individual and/or group)
- Regular exercise
- Antidepressant medication
- Engaging in meaningful activities
- Learning stress management strategies
- Social skills
- Positive environment and support strategies

Slide 14

Wellness Approach to Depression

- Pictures or video sequences
- Relaxation
- Guided Imagery
- Mindfulness
- Employment
- Recreation
- Exercise
- Friendship and dating
- Stress management

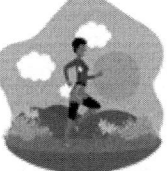

Slide 15

What symptoms of depression might look like for a person with IDD

Setup:	Set Off:	So I:	And I get or avoid:
Depression Not interested in previously motivating hobbies.	Prompted regarding "getting ready to leave/go out."	Ignore the cue and become aggressive if prompt is maintained.	Avoid going to out. activities and hobbies previously an incentive, but due to depression, formerly preferred events are no longer preferred.

Slide 16

BIPOLAR DISORDER

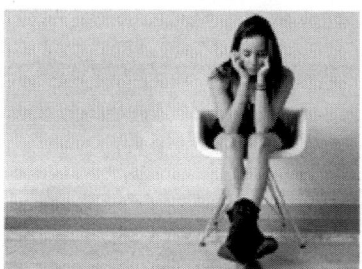

Image: freedigitalphotos.net/nenetus

Slide 17

Bipolar Disorder

- Persons with bipolar disorder may have periods of mania and periods of depression as well as normal moods.

- Bipolar disorder affects approximately 5.7 million adult Americans or about 2.8% of the U.S. population age 18 and older every year.

- Severe bipolar episodes of mania or depression may include psychotic symptoms such as hallucinations or delusions.

National Institute of Mental Health

Slide 18

Bipolar Disorder

Presentation in Someone with IDD

- Smiling, hugging or being affectionate with people who previously were not favored by the individual
- Boisterousness
- Over-reactivity to small incidents
- Extreme excitement
- Excessive laughing and giggling
- Self-injury associated with irritability
- Enthusiastic greeting of everyone

DM-ID-2

Slide 19

Bipolar Disorder

Presentation in Someone with IDD

- Behavioral challenges when prompted to go to try to sleep
- Constantly getting up at night
- Seems rested after not sleeping (i.e., not irritable due to lack of sleep as is common in depression)

DM-ID-2

Slide 20

Bipolar Disorder

Presentation in Someone with IDD

- Making improbable claims
- Dramatic physical presentation
- Dressing provocatively
- Demanding rewards
- Disorganized speech
- Thoughts not connected
- Quickly changing subjects

DM-ID-2

Slide 21

Bipolar Disorder

Presentation in Someone with IDD

- Increased singing
- Increased swearing
- Perseverative speech
- Screaming
- Frequent interrupting
- Nonverbal communication increases
- Increase in vocalizations

DM-ID-2

Slide 22

Bipolar Disorder

Presentation in Someone with IDD

- Decrease in work/task performance
- Leaving tasks incomplete
- Inability to settle (e.g., stay seated and focus on favorite TV show, stay seated through a complete activity when generally able to do so)

DM-ID-2

Slide 23

Bipolar Disorder

Presentation in Someone with IDD

- Pacing
- Negativism
- Working on many activities at once
- Fidgeting
- Aggression
- Rarely sits
- Increase in masturbation
- Giving away/spending money

DM-ID-2

Slide 24

Bipolar Disorder

Treatment Strategies

- Psychotherapy with a focus on understanding and managing the disorder
- Environmental and social modification (i.e., increase supervision to ensure safety)
- Positive support strategies
- Mood stabilizing and antidepressant medication

DM-ID- 2

MODULE 6

Slide 25

What symptoms of bipolar disorder might look like for a person with IDD

Setup:	Set Off:	So I:	And I get or avoid:
Bipolar cycling into manic phase. Not always a good sleeper. Not a lot of friends.	My DSP interrupts the activity I am busy with at 2 a.m. because it is loud (cleaning, laundry, playing guitar, watching TV).	I begin to scream and wake up my housemates.	My DSP allows me to return to activity since it is quieter than my screaming.

Slide 26

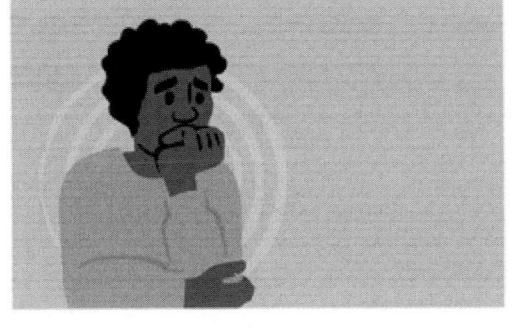

Slide 27

Anxiety Disorders

- Anxiety feels different for everyone. There are some outward signs of anxiety that we can observe. Other indicators of anxiety are internal symptoms that a person feels.
- Physical feelings of anxiety include rapid breathing, muscle tension, nausea, increased blood pressure, sweating, heart palpitations and chest pain.
- Other symptoms include restlessness, fatigue, irritability, sleep disturbances, difficulty concentrating, muscle tension, personality changes.

MODULE 6

Slide 28

Anxiety Disorders

Among the anxiety disorders listed in the DSM-5 are:

- **Generalized anxiety disorder:** This disorder involves excessive, anxiety or worry occurring more days than not for at least six months, about a number of events or activities.
- **Specific phobias:** Marked fear or anxiety about specific objects or situations, such as snakes, heights, flying, etc.
- **Social anxiety disorder:** Marked fear or anxiety about one or more social situations in which the person is exposed to possible scrutiny by others.
- **Panic disorder:** Recurrent, unexpected panic attacks.

APA, 2013

Slide 29

Anxiety Disorders

Presentation in Someone with IDD

- Restlessness
- Easily fatigued
- Difficulty concentrating
- Irritability
- Muscle tension
- Sleep disturbances
- Fear
- Avoidance

DM-ID-2

Slide 30

Anxiety Disorders

Anxiety and Repetitive Behavior

- Some anxiety disorders are accompanied by behaviors which are common in autism spectrum disorder (ASD) and other disorders.
- Many people, including individuals with ASD, engage in repetitive behaviors to help feel organized or comfortable.
- Compulsions are time-consuming and unhelpful behaviors. They interfere with other important and enjoyable areas of life. Behaviors are no longer functional or helpful if they cause distress rather than provide comfort.

MODULE 6

Slide 31

Anxiety Disorders

Treatment Strategies

- Psychotherapy with a focus on understanding and managing the disorder
- Environmental and social modification
- Social skill training
- Regular exercise
- Wellness-based approaches
- Learning stress management strategies
- Anti-anxiety medication

Hughes, 2006

Slide 32

What symptoms of anxiety might look like for a person with IDD

Setup:	Set Off:	So I:	And I get or avoid:
"I experience an anxiety disorder and autism."	Sees item "out of place" (e.g. thread on clothing, jars on a shelf, store display).	Charge at items or person to "fix" or rearrange, knocking down things in the process.	I fix the item out of place.
Low tolerance for "things out of place."			I feel relief and control over my environment.
Sensitive to noise and crowds.			
Poor verbal skills.			

Slide 33

PERSONALITY DISORDERS

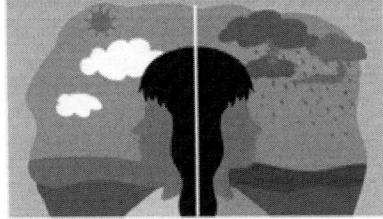

Slide 34

Personality Disorders

Personality disorders are mental health disorders characterized by inflexible and unhealthy patterns of thinking, feeling and behaving.

Symptoms include:

- Impulsivity with risk taking, spending, sexuality activity
- Overreliance on caregivers
- Mood swings
- Volatile relationship
- Social isolation
- Need for instant gratification
- Mistrust of others (especially strangers)
- Intense anxiety or irritability
- Poor impulse control

Slide 35

Personality Disorders

Among the different types of personality disorders listed in the DSM-5 are:

- **General Personality Disorder:** Enduring pattern of inner thoughts or behavior that deviates markedly from the expectations of the individual's culture.
- **Paranoid Personality Disorder:** Pervasive distrust or suspiciousness of others such that their behavior is interpreted as malevolent.
- **Dependent Personality Disorder:** Pervasive and excessive need to be taken care of that leads to submissive and clinging behavior and fear of separation.

APA, 2013

Slide 36

Personality Disorders

Presentation in Someone with IDD

- More reliant on caregivers than general population. Cultural sensitivities must also be considered.
- Frantic efforts to avoid real or imagined abandonment.
- Pattern of unstable and intense interpersonal relationships alternating between idealization and devaluation.
- Impulsivity in areas of spending, sexual activity, substance abuse, binge eating.
- Identity disturbance: markedly and persistently unstable self-image or sense of self.

DM-ID-2

M
O
D
U
L
E

6

Slide 37

Personality Disorders

Presentation in Someone with IDD

- Recurrent suicidal behavior, gestures, threats or self-mutilating behavior. Note: Self-injury can be a frequent problem for people with IDD and can be attributed to different causes.
- Irritability, intense episodic dysphoria/feeling of unease, anxiety usually lasting only a few hours.
- Chronic feelings of emptiness which may be difficult to express.

DM-ID-2

Slide 38

Personality Disorders

Treatment Strategies

- Individual or group therapy—cognitive and dialectical behavior therapy are most effective
- Environmental and social modification
- Social skill training
- Regular exercise
- Positive behavioral supports
- Psychotropic medication can be helpful for primary presenting symptoms
- Emotional regulation
- Learning stress management strategies/stress tolerance
- Positive identity development

Slide 39

What symptoms of borderline personality disorder might look like for a person with IDD

Setup:	Set Off:	So I:	And I get or avoid:
Borderline personality disorder.	Staff are arguing back and forth.	Make the divide between staff bigger escalating their argument.	I get to watch the conflict and drama that result.
Lots of staff turnover.			I am in the "starring role."
Live with roommates who are not good peer match, prefer company and role of staff.			
New manager creates conflict on the team.			

Slide 40

SCHIZOPHRENIA AND OTHER PSYCHOSIS

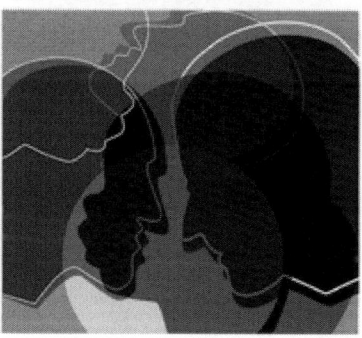

Slide 41

Psychosis

- The defining characteristics of psychosis are delusions, hallucinations and disorganized speech or behavior.

- Clinicians should be aware that any significant change in behavior can signify the possibility of psychosis (e.g., increase in self-injury, aggressive behavior or atypical behavior for the person).

DM-ID, 2007

Slide 42

Psychosis

Among the psychotic disorders listed in the DSM-5 are:

- Schizoaffective disorder
- Delusional disorder
- Schizophreniform disorder
- Substance/medication-induced psychotic disorder

APA, 2013

Slide 43

Psychosis

Presentation in Someone with IDD

- Delusions
- Hallucinations
- Disorganized speech
- Grossly disorganized behavior
- Negative symptoms (i.e., affect flattening, newly evidenced inability to speak, general lack of motivation or desire to pursue meaningful goals)

NOTE: Developmentally appropriate self-talk, imaginary friends, fantasy play and beliefs based on faulty learning can be confused with hallucinations and delusions.

DM-ID-2

Slide 44

Psychosis

Treatment Strategies

- Structure and consistency
- Social skills and stress management teaching
- Vocational training
- Positive support strategies
- Education regarding schizophrenia
- Recreation therapy
- Antipsychotic medication

Slide 45

What symptoms of psychosis might look like for a person with IDD...

Setup:	Set Off:	So I:	And I get or avoid:
Psychosis Lives with three other people with IDD.	Auditory hallucination at breakfast.	Yell back to "the voice."	Roommates take their coffee out to the porch.

MODULE 6

Slide 46

Indicators of a Mental Health Condition

- There is rapid onset, increase or change in behavior or symptoms
- There are changes in sleep or eating patterns
- There is a decrease in living skills or change in appearance or hygiene
- There is evidence of purposeful self-harm
- There are signs of hallucination or delusion
- There is co-occurring substance abuse
- The behavior/symptoms occurs across all environments, not just one specific setting

M
O
D
U
L
E

6

Post-test

Module VI: Signs and Symptoms of Mental Illness

_____ 1. What is the difference between anxiety people commonly feel in everyday life and having an anxiety disorder?
(a) Whether people see a therapist
(b) There is no difference
(c) Whether the anxiety interferes with quality of life
(d) If the person takes medication

_____ 2. Which factor(s) can complicate diagnosis of mental health disorders in people with IDD?
(a) People with IDD may have narrow communication that can limit their ability to describe their symptoms
(b) People with IDD may experience symptoms of mental health disorders differently
(c) The symptoms a person is experiencing may be connected to a known IDD diagnosis, when there may actually be another condition
(d) All of the above

_____ 3. True or false: Depression is not diagnosed as quickly for people with IDD as for the general population as onset tends to be more insidious and changes in baseline are not as apparent.

_____ 4. _____ refers to the process of attributing all an individual's symptoms to a known condition.
(a) Assessment
(b) Diagnostic overshadowing
(c) Polypharmacy
(d) Screening

_____ 5. True or false: A person with bipolar disorder will show cycling moods (periods of mania and periods of depression) over the course of days or hours.

_____ 6. This disorder involves excessive anxiety or worry occurring more days than not for at least six months, about a number of events or activities:
(a) Phobia
(b) Generalized anxiety disorder
(c) Panic disorder
(d) Obsessive-compulsive disorder

_____ 7. _____ cause difficulty perceiving and relating to situations and people, including oneself.

(a) Personality disorders

(b) Mood disorders

(c) Phobias

(d) Compulsions

_____ 8. Psychosis may present in someone with IDD with which of the following symptoms?

(a) Delusions

(b) Hallucinations

(c) Disorganized speech

(d) All of the above

_____ 9. Which is an example of a wellness strategy to help manage anxiety?

(a) Avoiding work when feeling nervous

(b) Skipping a party where you don't know many people

(c) Staying awake all night and worrying about a test the next day

(d) Attending weekly yoga classes with a friend

_____ 10. Which is the greatest indicator that behaviors may indicate an underlying mental health condition?

(a) The behavior never occurs when the person is at work

(b) The behavior occurs less frequently if the person eats breakfast

(c) The behavior occurs in all environments/across settings

(d) The behavior is only observed at home

MODULE 6

Supplemental Materials

Module VI: Signs and Symptoms of Mental Illness

Obtaining an accurate mental health diagnosis remains very challenging. Recognizing mental health conditions in people with IDD can be complicated by several factors.

In your experience, what are some signs or behaviors you may observe in a person with IDD who presents with the conditions listed below?

Depression	
Anxiety disorder	
Bipolar disorder	

Understanding behavior is an important part of recognizing indicators of a mental health condition. When we understand the underlying causes of behavior and symptoms, we can address them in a more meaningful way.

Use the grid below to consider how mental health symptoms may impact the behavior you observe.

How symptoms of a mental health condition may present for a person with IDD:

Setup:	Set Off:	So I:	And I get or avoid:
Symptoms	Trigger	Behavior	Outcome

Tools for Tracking Symptoms and Behavior Change

Use the checklist below to help gather more information about someone you know/support who may be exhibiting signs and symptoms. Provide more information where needed.

Indicators of a mental health condition	Notes
☐ There is rapid onset, increase or change in behavior or symptoms	
☐ There are changes in sleep or eating patterns	
☐ There is a decrease in living skills or change in appearance or hygiene	
☐ There is evidence of purposeful self-harm	
☐ There are signs of hallucination or delusion	
☐ There is co-occurring substance abuse	
☐ The behavior/symptom occurs across all environments, not just one specific setting	

M
O
D
U
L
E

6

Psychiatric Symptoms and Behavior Checklist

http://iddtoolkit.vkcsites.org/wp-content/uploads/PsychSymptomsBehChecklist.pdf

MODULE 6

Psychiatric Symptoms and Behavior Checklist	Name: _____ DOB ___/___/___

Checklist can be completed by primary care provider, or by caregiver and reviewed by provider

Please mark the list below:
- No symptoms--0
- Mild symptoms occasionally--1
- Mild symptoms some of the time--2
- Major symptoms some of the time--3
- Major symptoms all of the time--4

Symptoms and behaviors	BASELINE [1] Mark if usually present	NEW Mark if recent onset	COMMENTS If new onset or increased
Anxiety-related			
Anxiety			
Panic			
Phobias			
Obsessive thoughts			
Compulsive behaviors			
Rituals/routines			
Other			
Mood-related			
Agitation			
Irritability			
Aggression			
Self-injurious behavior			
Depressed mood			
Loss of interest • Unhappy/miserable • Under-activity			
Sleep issues			
Eating pattern			
Appetite			
Weight (provide details)			
Elevated mood			
Intrusiveness			
Hypersexuality			
Other			
Psychotic-related [2]			
Psychotic and psychotic-like symptoms (e.g., self talk, delusions, hallucinations)			
Movement-related			
Catatonia ('stuck')			
Tics			
Stereotypies (repetitive movements or utterances)			
ADHD-related or Mood Disorder			
Inattention			
Hyperactivity			
Impulsivity			
Dementia-related			
Concentration			
Memory			
Other			
Other			
Alcohol misuse			
Drug abuse			
Sexual issues/problems			
Psychosomatic complaints			

[1] Establish usual baseline i.e., behaviors and daily functioning before onset of concerns. [2] Use caution when interpreting psychotic-like symptoms and behaviors in patients with IDD. These may be associated with anxiety (or other circumstances) rather than a psychotic disorder.

Module VII

Positive Support
Strategies and Wellness

Pre-test

Module VII: Positive Support Strategies and Wellness

_____ 1. Which of the following is an example of positive behavior support (PBS)?
    (a) Overcorrection following property destruction
    (b) Teaching conversation skills
    (c) Toothbrushing goals
    (d) Using the Whately Principle to craft a reward scheme that will generalize

_____ 2. Which is a reason that inappropriate behavior is difficult to change?
    (a) It probably works for the person based on their history
    (b) It makes sense to the person
    (c) Both are true
    (d) Neither is true

_____ 3. Which of the following is not something PBS considers?
    (a) Quality of life
    (b) Effective consequence strategies
    (c) Learning history
    (d) Skill-building

_____ 4. When starting a conversation, it is a good idea to:
    (a) Start with limit-setting statements
    (b) Remind the person you are in charge
    (c) All of the above
    (d) None of the above

_____ 5. How might one effectively adapt an environment that causes problems for a person?
    (a) Tell the person to ignore whatever is bothering them
    (b) Change the troubling feature, such as choosing a more pleasant tone for an alarm
    (c) There is no effective way to change an environment
    (d) Use Hastur's Behavioral Model as an analysis method

_____ 6. What is the purpose of relaxation?
    (a) Supporting a person to be calmer
    (b) Supporting a person to handle stress better
    (c) It is a simple way to improve quality of life
    (d) All of the above

M O D U L E 7

_____ 7. Which is an example of Feil's Validation Strategy?
(a) Asking what a person's favorite beverage is if they are upset over losing their drink
(b) Reminding the person that their roommates haven't ever stolen things
(c) Correcting misperceptions
(d) All of the above

_____ 8. Wellness interventions are:
(a) A good starting point for interventions
(b) Unlikely to make things worse
(c) Both (a) and (b) are true
(d) Neither (a) nor (b) is true

_____ 9. Which of the following is not a wellness intervention?
(a) Improving relaxation
(b) Promoting reading
(c) Natural consequences
(d) Nature walks

_____ 10. PRN stands for:
(a) Per Resources Nullification
(b) Pro Re Nata
(c) Pax Riley Non
(d) Pickman Rand Nephren

Slide 1

Module VII

**Positive Support
Strategies and Wellness**

Slide 2

Learning Objectives

- Discuss five principles for achieving a therapeutic relationship.
- Name three special considerations when conducting therapy with people who have IDD/MI.
- Describe the main characteristics and components of positive behavior supports.

Slide 3

In this module, we will discuss the following advanced support strategies:

1. Positive behavior supports
2. Communication tone
3. Environmental
4. Choice and self-determination
5. Relaxation techniques
6. Verbal strategies

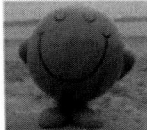

Slide 4

Positive Behavior Support

Positive Behavior Support (PBS) involves the changing situations and events that people with problem behaviors experience in order to reduce the likelihood of their occurrence and increase social, personal and professional quality in their lives.

Carr & Sidener, 2002

Slide 5

What Does PBS Consider?

- Values about the rights and dignity of people who have disabilities and self-determination
- Practical science about how learning and behavior change occur
- Biomedical concerns
- Lifestyle concerns
- Changes in systems of support
- Team-based approaches

Carr & Sidener, 2002

Slide 6

Considerations

- Decrease negative behaviors
- Support appropriate behavior
- Focus on improving environment, not "fixing" people
- Quality-of-life enhancement
- Increase learning and independence
- Successful input and collaboration from those closest to the person and the person themselves
- Cooperation across disciplines

Carr & Sidener, 2002

Slide 7

Components of a PBS Approach

- Functional assessment

- Comprehensive intervention

- Focus on quality of life and wellness

Carr & Sidener, 2002

Slide 8

1. **The Importance of Communication:**

Setting the tone

- Begin your interaction socially.

- Use a non-demanding

  approach.

- Give choices

  whenever possible.

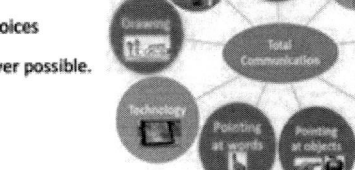

Hughes, 2006

Slide 9

2. **Environmental Contributors to Problem Behaviors**

  - Important to evaluate the environment

  - Look for things that might be contributing to, or triggering, problem behaviors

    NOTE: Important to look at environment from the person's perspective.

Griffiths, Gardner & Nugent, 1998

Slide 10

Exercise

Activity: Consider environmental contributors and solutions for the following behaviors:

- Eduardo has been removing his clothes in the classroom. This only occurs in the winter months when he is often wearing sweaters.

- Laura will scream and bite her hand at the kitchen table during meal times.

- Angel bangs his head against the window on the school bus. Recently, the bus changed routes, so this changed the order of his pick-up and the location of his seat on the bus.

Slide 11

---

3. Providing Choice and Self-Determination

Guiding Principle: Choice has positive benefits:

- Increases community integration
- Increases adaptive behavior
- Improves overall quality of life
- Decreases problem behavior

Slide 12

---

4. Relaxation Techniques

The purpose is to help the individual self manage and reduce stress, tension and/or angry feelings.

Relaxation strategies distract the person from the source of the stress and place focus on appropriate behavior.

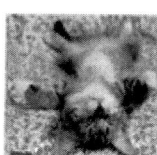

Hughes, 2006

M
O
D
U
L
E

7

Slide 13

Let's Practice Together
PMR: Progressive Muscle Relaxation

Sit in a relaxed position.
Focus on yourself and on achieving relaxation in specific body muscles.
Tune out all other thoughts.
Squeeze fists together tightly. Slowly count to five and release.
Shrug your shoulders up to your ears for five seconds. Relax.
Arch your back off the floor for five seconds. Relax.
Squeeze legs tightly and slowly count to five and release.
Repeat for other body parts that are tense.
Avoid body parts that are sore or uncomfortable.

Slide 14

What Do You Find Relaxing?

Activity: Think of an activity that you find relaxing:
- Playing an instrument? Listening to music? Attending concert?
- Taking a walk or hiking?
- Word puzzles or board games?
- Dancing, aerobics, jogging or other exercise?
- Watching TV? Going to the movies?
- Cooking, reading, sewing, scrapbooking?

Using your interest and familiarity, design an activity for an individual or group in the setting where you work that promotes proactive relaxation opportunities. Build the most successful ideas into your regular routine!

Slide 15

5. Verbal Strategy
- Verbal techniques can help an individual feel acknowledged and supported.
- Verbal techniques can be used by direct care staff as well as clinical staff.
  - a. Validating
  - b. Exploring
  - c. Problem-solving

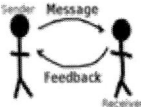

Hughes, 2008

Slide 16

5. a) Validating

Validating involves confirming the person's emotions.

An example of this is shown in the following scenario:

Jack: "Everybody around here hates me!"

Staff: "It sounds as though you are pretty angry."

Hughes, 2006

Slide 17

5. b) Validating and Exploring

Validating and exploring can be combined and involve encouraging the individual to further explain whatever it is the individual is trying to communicate.

An example of this is shown in the following scenario:

Jack: "Everybody around here hates me!"

Staff: "It sounds like you are pretty angry. Can you tell me what you are so mad about?"

Hughes, 2006

Slide 18

5. c) Problem-Solving

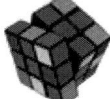

- Identify the nature of the problem from the client's point of view.

- Explore alternative solutions to the problem.

- Implement the best alternative solution.

Hughes, 2006

Slide 19

Exercise: Verbal Strategies

You are working with a woman named Lorraine who believes that one of her staff or roommates steals her clothes from the laundry room. As a result she will no longer wash her clothes, wearing the same soiled outfits to work every day. When you approach Lorraine about this, she screams and yells about people stealing and not trusting anyone to help her.

Activity: Consider the three verbal strategies reviewed on the prior slides to help Lorraine feel acknowledged and supported in reaching a productive and positive outcome.

Slide 20

Effective Communication Strategies

There are certain communication techniques that can be very helpful in de-escalating situations. These include:

1. Active listening

2. Empathetic responses

3. Maintain a nonjudgmental attitude

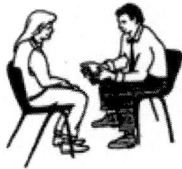

McGilvery & Sweetland, 2011

Slide 21

Effective Communication Strategies

4. Recognize and avoid power struggles

5. Watch your posture and body language

6. Validate feelings

7. Put the choices back to the person

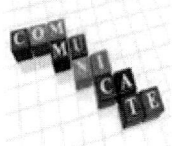

McGilvery & Sweetland, 2011

Slide 22

Crisis Prevention and Planning

By addressing environmental, biological, psychological and social factors that may contribute to problem behavior, staff may be able to assist the person to cope, maintain control of his/her own behavior and learn positive, productive ways that address the function of the behavior.

Slide 23

Nonverbal De-Escalation Strategies

1. Monitor your body position and body language.

2. Avoid physically putting yourself in harm's way.

3. Maintain a demeanor of calmness, neutrality and confidence.

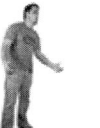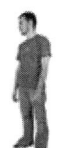

McGilvery & Sweetland, 2011

Slide 24

Verbal De-Escalation Strategies

1. Use a calm tone of voice.

2. Use reflective listening.

3. Avoid threatening punishment.

4. Avoid power struggles.

5. Do not ignore escalations of behaviors that could lead to severe behaviors.

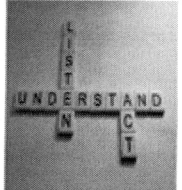

McGilvery & Sweetland, 2011

M
O
D
U
L
E

7

Slide 25

Verbal De-Escalation Strategies

6. Change staffing if necessary.

7. Affirm that you understand.

8. Change the subject if it appears to agitate the person more to talk about it (e.g., offer a drink of water, bring up an topic that interests him or her such as sporting event or TV program).

McGilvery & Sweetland, 2011

Slide 26

Verbal De-Escalation Strategies

9. Change aspects of the environment.

10. Set limits by reminding the person of the choices and outcomes but do so in a firm, fair manner and with a non-emotional tone of voice.

11. Remind the individual of the desirable consequences of choosing a positive behavior as opposed to a problem behavior. Then remind the persons of the undesirable consequences that can occur if they engage in the problem behavior.

McGilvery & Sweetland, 2011

Slide 27

PROMOTING MENTAL WELLNESS

Slide 28

**Promoting Mental Wellness:
How Do We Often Look at Supports?**

- When we think about how to support people with Intellectual or Developmental Disabilities (IDD) who are having a difficult time, we think about how the disability impacts the person's life or we look at what support to use to make things better.

- For people with challenging behavior (also referred to as *interfering* behavior), we often consider why the person has difficulties. In other words, we are often focused on what is "wrong" with a person's life.

Slide 29

**Promoting Mental Wellness:
What Is Mental Wellness?**

- Sometimes we miss asking whether people are "well."

- Are we thinking about how to support the person in engaging in a healthy lifestyle that will promote mental wellness and having a good life?

Slide 30

**Promoting Mental Wellness:
How Do We Promote Wellness?**

- There are day-to-day factors that make up what we call *wellness*. Think about this in our own lives; when we are not feeling ourselves or feeling stressed, we may have many ways of coping.

- We also have our own ways of living a life that is meaningful to us.

- We can take actions such as: taking a new and better job, having the ability to be spontaneous and splurge, take a day for ourselves, enjoy a relaxing bath, hit the gym or get lost in in our favorite hobby.

Slide 31

Promoting Wellness as Part of Supporting a Person with IDD?

- Mental wellness is an important part of a positive supports framework.

- JoAnn Cannon offers an evidence-based way to think about wellness (Cannon, 2005)

Slide 32

Promoting Mental Wellness
How Do We Promote Wellness?

JoAnn Cannon's 15 Factors Related to Wellness
(*Enhancing the Good*, 2005)

Contact with nature	Experienced creativity
Optimism	Balanced nutrition
Work satisfaction	Goal accomplishment
Economic essentials	Intellectual stimulation
Coping with stress	Rest and sleep
Spirit awareness	Time and space alone
Positive self-image	Physical prowess
Fulfilling relationships	

Slide 33

Exercise

Pick one of the wellness areas identified by Dr. Cannon and identify three different things you could do to assist a person with IDD to have a better life in that area.

This can be done individually or in groups.

MODULE 7

Slide 34

Are Wellness Factors Included in Your Support Plans?

- Where would they fit?
  - Behavior support plan?
  - General support planning document?

- What data would you collect?

Slide 35

How Might Wellness Be Considered?

- Consider the "15 Factors of Wellness" when creating support plans.
  - Does the person have a chance to engage in each of these factors?
  - Can we provide assistance in working to better the person's life with respect to these factors?
- If somebody is having challenging behaviors, look at wellness as part of the assessment process.
- If a team of care providers looks at that list and doesn't know how the person is doing on them, the first step is to learn more about how the person sees his or her life.
- Support wellness to ensure that you are not only meeting the person's immediate needs, but also the things that will increase the quality of life.

Slide 36

RATIONAL APPROACH TO

PSYCHOPHARMACOLOGY

Slide 37

MYTH: MEDICATION TREATMENT IS USED TO CONTROL MALADAPTIVE BEHAVIORS

Premise:
Medication-based therapies directly affect behavior.

Reality:
Behaviors such as self-injury and aggression are too nonspecific to be considered as direct targets for drug therapy.

Treatment implications:
The appropriate targets for medication therapy are the changes in neurophysiological function that mediate behavior associated with psychiatric disorders.

Slide 38

Medication Treatment

Pharmacotherapy is therapeutic and may be the first choice treatment for some psychiatric disorders:

- Major depression
- Mania states
- Schizophrenia

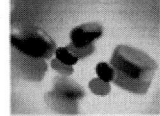

Medication treatment should be diagnostically related to a DSM-5 diagnostic and treatment guideline or the DM-ID.

Slide 39

General Best Practices in Psychopharmacology

- An assessment of mental illness should guide intervention and findings should be shared.
- Medication and non-medication intervention should be used together.
- A written treatment plan should be developed and shared.
- Generally, one medication at a time should be prescribed.

M O D U L E 7

Slide 40

Necessary Communication

- The prescriber should share all relevant information about the medication in understandable language.
- The prescriber should dictate what information is needed back to make good decisions about medication management.
- Side effects monitoring should be established.

Slide 41

PRN Medication

- Some medications can be offered as needed, which is termed "pro re nata" or PRN.
- The prescriber should give detailed information about when PRNs should be given and monitor how much they are used.
- Be aware that there might be rules about PRN medication in some areas.

Slide 42

Putting It All Together

Activity: Develop a blueprint wellness plan for someone you support. Consider the support strategies reviewed in this chapter that would apply to him/her.

Tips:

- Identity the person's strengths and interests.
- Consider the person's diagnosis and mental health needs.
- Promote relaxation opportunities.
- Anticipate challenges and be prepared with de-escalation and validation strategies.
- Build in ways to help the person feel good about him/herself and develop positive identify.
- Monitor behavior and medication information.

M
O
D
U
L
E

7

Post-test

Module VII: Positive Support Strategies and Wellness

_____ 1. Which of the following is an example of positive behavior support (PBS)?
(a) Overcorrection following property destruction
(b) Teaching conversation skills
(c) Toothbrushing goals
(d) Using the Whately Principle to craft a reward scheme that will generalize

_____ 2. Which is a reason that inappropriate behavior is difficult to change?
(a) It probably works for the person based on their history
(b) It makes sense to the person
(c) Both are true
(d) Neither is true

_____ 3. Which of the following is not something PBS considers?
(a) Quality of life
(b) Effective consequence strategies
(c) Learning history
(d) Skill-building

_____ 4. When starting a conversation, it is a good idea to:
(a) Start with limit-setting statements
(b) Remind the person you are in charge
(c) All of the above
(d) None of the above

_____ 5. How might one effectively adapt an environment that causes problems for a person?
(a) Tell the person to ignore whatever is bothering them
(b) Change the troubling feature, such as choosing a more pleasant tone for an alarm
(c) There is no effective way to change an environment
(d) Use Hastur's Behavioral Model as an analysis method

_____ 6. What is the purpose of relaxation?
(a) Supporting a person to be calmer
(b) Supporting a person to handle stress better
(c) It is a simple way to improve quality of life
(d) All of the above

M
O
D
U
L
E

7

_____ 7. Which is an example of Feil's Validation Strategy?
(a) Asking what a person's favorite beverage is if they are upset over losing their drink
(b) Reminding the person that their roommates haven't ever stolen things
(c) Correcting misperceptions
(d) All of the above

_____ 8. Wellness interventions are:
(a) A good starting point for interventions
(b) Unlikely to make things worse
(c) Both (a) and (b) are true
(d) Neither (a) nor (b) is true

_____ 9. Which of the following is not a wellness intervention?
(a) Improving relaxation
(b) Promoting reading
(c) Natural consequences
(d) Nature walks

_____ 10. PRN stands for:
(a) Per Resources Nullification
(b) Pro Re Nata
(c) Pax Riley Non
(d) Pickman Rand Nephren

MODULE

7

Supplemental Materials

Module VII: Positive Support Strategies and Wellness

Positive Behavior Supports

In this module, we talked a lot about how positive supports come from values around how to support people with disabilities. What are your values about how to support people with disabilities who also have behavior support needs?

_____

_____

What do you think you should do as a care provider when you see a person making a mistake, such as dating a person who is taking advantage of them?

_____

_____

What would you do if a friend was dating a person who is taking advantage of them?

_____

_____

What would you do if a family member was dating a person who is taking advantage of them?

_____

_____

Conversation Starters

What are 10 good ways to start a positive conversation with somebody? Remember that this module has many good tips!

1. _____

2. _____

3. _____

4. _____

5. _____

6. _____

7. _____

8. _____

9. _____

10. _____

M
O
D
U
L
E

7

The Environment

Please make a list of things that bother you in an environment. We will give you the first one.

1. <u>Car alarms in the middle of the night</u>

2. _____

3. _____

4. _____

5. _____

6. _____

7. _____

8. _____

9. _____

10. _____

Are there things on this list that probably wouldn't bother other people? Put a **star** by them. For example, loud chewing sounds bother some people but not others.

Now **circle** the ones that might bother a person you support.

Relaxation

In this module, we discuss the need for coping and relaxation. List 10 things you do to relax.

1. _____

2. _____

3. _____

4. _____

5. _____

6. _____

7. _____

8. _____

9. _____

10. _____

What do you do to relax when you are really stressed?

_____

_____

What helps calm you when you are really worried?

_____

_____

M
O
D
U
L
E

7

Crisis Planning

What do you think are the most important parts of responding to crises?

_____

_____

What has helped most in your experience?

_____

_____

An old saying goes, "Once you are in a power struggle, you have already lost." What are some ways you can avoid power struggles?

_____

_____

Mental Wellness

What makes you feel mentally well?

_____

_____

When do you feel at your best?

_____

_____

What do you do to help people you support feel mentally well?

_____

_____

**M
O
D
U
L
E

7**

Psychopharmacology

Do you know about the medications and side effects for people you support?

_____

_____

How might you learn more about the medications taken by the people you support?

_____

_____

M
O
D
U
L
E

7

Module VIII

Crisis Prevention and Intervention: Reducing Risk

Pre-test

Module VIII: Crisis Prevention and Intervention: Reducing Risk

_____ 1. _____ refers to strategies and responses used once signs of crisis are already present.
(a) Behavior modification
(b) Crisis intervention
(c) Crisis prevention
(d) Informed consent

_____ 2. True or false: Most crises can be prevented or interrupted before harm occurs.

_____ 3. A crisis plan should:
(a) Outline what constitutes a crisis for the person and which actions to take to prevent and respond to crises
(b) Include a list of PRN medications to keep administering until the person is calm
(c) Only be used if 911 or other emergency services are called
(d) Require authorization from a psychiatrist

_____ 4. _____ are lifestyle measures (such as relationships, routine and wellness) that minimize the impact of a crisis or prevent a behavior from escalating.
(a) Symptoms
(b) Protective factors
(c) Risk factors
(d) Triggers

_____ 5. Factors that can precipitate a crisis include:
(a) Grief and loss
(b) Medication changes or side effects
(c) Unemployment
(d) All of the above
(e) Only (a) and (b)

_____ 6. Crises can be prevented:
(a) By keeping people isolated from the community and each other
(b) After the first time a person goes to the emergency department
(c) By addressing environmental, biological, psychological and social factors that contribute to behavior
(d) With enough medication

MODULE 8

_____ 7. What are some challenges with the current crisis system for people with IDD?
(a) There is a lack of psychiatric services for both adults and children with IDD
(b) Lack of available community programs leads to overutilization of emergency resources
(c) People with IDD are at risk of losing homes or jobs following inpatient admission
(d) All of the above

_____ 8. True or false: Risk assessment used to evaluate a crisis for the general population is not an applicable tool for people with IDD.

_____ 9. During the _____ phase of crisis intervention, helpful responses include supportive verbal techniques, maintaining safety, providing distraction and validation.
(a) Baseline
(b) Prevention
(c) Escalation
(d) Resolution

_____ 10. _____ is based on the idea that negative outcomes result from faulty systems, rather than ineffective people.
(a) Collaboration
(b) Triage
(c) Training
(d) Inclusion

M
O
D
U
L
E

8

MODULE 8

Slide 1

Module VIII

**Crisis Prevention and Intervention:
Reducing Risk**

Slide 2

Learning Objectives

- Recognize why people with IDD/MI are more likely to experience conditions that can lead to a crisis.
- Recognize how unmet mental health needs can contribute to a crisis.
- Identify components of safe, effective crisis prevention and intervention strategies.

Slide 3

What Is a Crisis?

- Crisis is defined as a situation when support needs for a person are greater than what the setting can offer.
- Crises might occur when a person's level of behavioral health challenges overwhelm a home or job site.
- Instability in a home setting may reduce supports available.
- Support needs include health care.

Slide 4

Crisis Intervention and Prevention

A crisis occurs when a person is feeling threatened, suffers sudden loss or change or cannot access skills or resources.

Behavior is an attempt to meet a need; it has meaning for the person. Repeated problem behavior should not be looked at as a crisis. Inadequate or improper supports contribute to ongoing unmet needs.

Slide 5

Impact of Crisis

- Consider the risk factors (history of behaviors) and protective factors (social supports, community) that determine how severe a crisis can become.

- Strengthening these protective factors for a person prior to a potential crisis is a crucial prevention step.

- Trauma can trigger or exacerbate a crisis.

Slide 6

Being Proactive

- Use behavior and health information to help prevent or prepare for a crisis.

- Describe how to recognize patterns of escalating behaviors or symptoms and ways to intervene as early as possible.

MODULE 8

Slide 7

Crisis Identification

- What does crisis mean to you?
- Who's really having the crisis?
- Ongoing monitoring and observation
- The earlier we recognize the problem, the better.
- It helps to know the person well, what his/her needs are, patterns of behavior, identify precursors of escalation, recognize and document response strategies.

MODULE 8

Slide 8

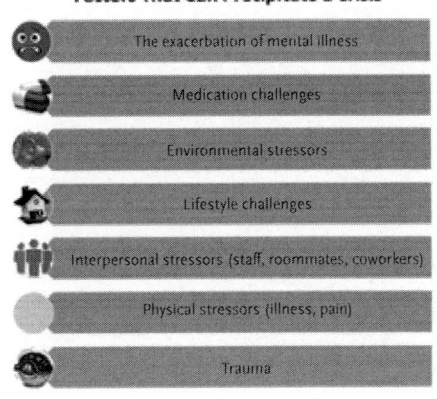

Factors That Can Precipitate a Crisis

- The exacerbation of mental illness
- Medication challenges
- Environmental stressors
- Lifestyle challenges
- Interpersonal stressors (staff, roommates, coworkers)
- Physical stressors (illness, pain)
- Trauma

Slide 9

More Factors That Can Precipitate a Crisis

- Inadequate behavior supports
- Grief and loss
- Effects of medication
- Transition
- Loss or change in services
- Diagnosis
- Unemployment
- Poverty

Cheplic, 2016

Slide 10

**The Need for IDD
Crisis Services**

- When a behavioral health crisis occurs, the primary means of response are to take an individual to the emergency department or call 911.

- Law enforcement may become involved at the individual's home or job or in the community.

- Hospitals may provide medication to calm the individual and send them home, may use restraints, may not screen for pain, GI symptoms, medication side effects, etc.

Cheplic, 2016

Slide 11

Understanding Behavior

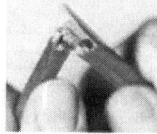

- Repeated problem behavior should not be seen as a crisis.

- By addressing environmental, biological, psychological and social factors that contribute to problem behavior, crises can be prevented or interrupted.

- The continued need to consider emergency/crisis services is an indicator that behavior or treatment plans aren't working.

Slide 12

Recognizing Signs and Providing Supports

The following example is an illustration of a scenario that, when handled poorly, resulted in a crisis:

Kyle was fired from his job yesterday. At breakfast, he tells his roommate he is going to get even with his boss when the time is right.

What are your next steps?

M
O
D
U
L
E

8

Slide 13

Crisis Intervention and Prevention

- What immediate steps should be taken to ensure safety?

- What factors contributed to this incident?

- How could this crisis have been prevented?

- What could each of the players have done differently?

- What are the next steps in planning Bill's behavior supports?

Slide 14

Crisis Response

- Provide visual aids and include individuals in planning to help reduce uncertainty and anxiety.

- Recognize that repeating questions or ruminating on a topic may be a coping strategy for the person.

- Setting clear expectations in advance helps support respectful communication and recognize a problem as early as possible.

Slide 15

The Big Picture: Reducing Crises

- Establish environments that reduce/prevent crisis.
- View behaviors as indicators of where assistance is needed.
- Support ongoing wellness and relaxation opportunities for all individuals, with extra emphasis on mental health supports for those with a psychiatric diagnosis.
- Make activities engaging, supportive, interactive, person-centered, choice-driven and safe.
- Provide immediate crisis prevention and response services in the community.

Slide 16

Challenges with Current System

- Community has a lack of psychiatric services for both adults and children with IDD/MI.

- Overutilization of community emergency resources due to lack of community crisis programs.

- Potential loss of residence or employment when an individual is admitted to a hospital or goes to jail.

Slide 17

Bio-Psycho-Social Model: What is Precipitating the Crises?

Bio-psycho-social framework: an approach to describing and explaining how *biological, psychological* and *social* factors combine and interact to influence physical and mental health

Psychological
- learning
- emotions
- thinking
- attitudes
- memory
- perceptions
- beliefs
- stress management strategies

Biological
- genetic predisposition
- neurochemistry
- effect of medications
- immune response
- HPA axis
- fight-flight response
- physiological responses

Social
- social support
- family background
- interpersonal relationships
- cultural traditions
- medical care
- socio-economic status
- poverty
- physical exercise
- biofeedback

Adapted from Griffiths & Gardner, 2002

Slide 18

Crisis Prevention and Management Plan

Slide 19

**Components
of a Crisis Prevention Plan**

A crisis prevention plan is intended to be an informative and helpful planning tool for consumers, families and providers to aid in the early detection of and effective intervention during an emergent situation.

Slide 20

Crisis Intervention and Prevention

Stage of Behavior	Response
Baseline: Normal, calm	Positive approaches: clear communication, structure, routine, sensory needs
Prevention (early warning signs, i.e. anxiety or agitation)	Be supportive, modify environment to meet needs & decrease stressors (de-escalation strategies)
Escalation (defensive or resistant, verbal threats)	Reduce risk, verbal techniques, maintain safety, distraction, validation
Crisis (aggression, risk of harm to self or others)	Continue positive interaction, safe response strategies, i.e., remind the patient with DD of pre-established boundaries; remind him/her about outcomes and next steps without threatening
Resolution and calming	Re-establish routines and re-establish rapport; prevent future escalation

porticonetwork.ca CAMH

Slide 21

**Components
of a Crisis Prevention Plan**

- Presenting problem
- Early warning signs (precipitants)
- What has helped in the past?
- What action is helpful?
- What action is not helpful?
- Summary

Slide 22

**Components
of a Crisis Prevention Plan**

- What needs does the behavior seem to meet?
- List known antecedents/triggers
- List protective factors: What is valuable and important to him/her?
- Communication skills: Describe the primary methods used by this person to communicate (vocal speech, signs, gestures, communication books, electronic devices or behavior etc.).

Slide 23

**Components
of a Crisis Prevention Plan**

- It identifies a person's response patterns to manage a crisis when it occurs.

- The crisis prevention and management plan is best developed by a team.

First Response to Victims of Crime, 2008

Slide 24

**Components
of a Crisis Prevention Plan**

- Outlines safe and effective crisis intervention strategies when necessary.

- Describes how to recognize patterns of escalating behaviors.

M
O
D
U
L
E

8

Slide 25

**Components
of a Crisis Prevention Plan**

- Purpose is to help prevent or prepare for a crisis.

- Includes specific needs and triggers of individuals supported.

First Response to Victims of Crime, 2008

Slide 26

**Components
of a Crisis Prevention Plan**

Describe the behavior in operational terms (specify how the behavior is performed):

Behavior	Operational Description

Slide 27

**Crisis Prevention
and Management Plan**

Stage of Observed Behavior	Recommended Caregiver Responses
Stage 1: Normal, calm behavior	Use positive approaches, encourage usual routines.
Stage 2: Prevention (Identify early warning signs that signal increasing stress or anxiety.)	Be supportive, modify environment to meet needs (Identify de-escalation strategies that are helpful for this person with DD).
Stage 3: Escalation (Identify signs that the person is escalating to a possible behavior crisis.)	Be directive (use verbal direction & modeling), continue to modify environment to meet needs, ensure safety.
Stage 4: Crisis (Risk of harm to self, others or environment or seriously disruptive behavior, e.g., acting out.)	Use safety and crisis response strategies.
Stage 5: Post-crisis resolution and calming	Re-establish routines and re-establish rapport.

Surrey Place Centre, 2011

Slide 28

**Risk Assessment Tool
for Behavioral Crisis**

Utilize risk assessments applicable to the general population. Take into account how the person's developmental disabilities affect both risks and protective factors. Note whether recent changes have occurred in any risk or protective factors.

Flag all areas where there are risk issues. Also consider factors that may protect from harm.

Adapted from Surrey Place Centre, 2011

Slide 29

**Risk Assessment Tool
for Behavioral Crisis**

Risk Area	Person – Risk Factors	Caregivers / Environment Assessment
Harm to self	Is the person verbalizing suicidal thoughts or intent? Is there evidence of suicidal behaviors, poor judgment or mental illness? Is there a history of suicidal or para-suicidal behavior? Is the patient unable to identify reasons to keep on living? Is the patient engaging in, or is there evidence of, self-harm? Is the patient verbalizing intent to self-harm? Does the person have a history of self-harm? Is the person unable to care for self? Is the person unwilling to accept support from others? Is there evidence of neglect & behaviors that put the patient at risk?	Is a means available for the person to commit suicide? Are means available for individual to harm self? Are caregivers able to supervise and protect the person? Are others available and able to assist in the person's care?

Adapted from Surrey Place Centre, 2011

Slide 30

**Risk Assessment Tool
for Behavioral Crisis**

Risk Area	Person – Risk Factors	Caregivers / Environment Assessment
Victimization or exploitation	Is the patient being victimized or exploited? Has the person been victimized or exploited in the past? Is the person unable to protect self? Does the person lack insight into possible dangers of the situation? Has the patient failed to show evidence that he/she would ask for help? Has the person been unable to get help or protection from others in the past?	Are caregivers able to supervise and protect the person?

Adapted from Surrey Place Centre, 2011

MODULE 8

Slide 31

Risk Assessment Tool
for Behavioral Crisis

Risk Area	Person – Risk Factors	Caregivers / Environment Assessment
Harm to others	Is the person verbalizing intent to harm others? Is the person making physical gestures about hurting others? Has the person caused physical harm to others? Does the person have sufficient mobility and strength to potentially harm others? Does the patient's aggression/harmful behavior tend to escalate quickly and/or unpredictably?	Are there vulnerable individuals in the setting who cannot protect themselves? Can caregivers recognize cues and intervene safely? Can the person be supervised safely in current setting without caregivers being at risk of harm while trying to prevent harm to others?

Adapted from Surrey Place Centre, 2011

Slide 32

Risk Assessment Tool
for Behavioral Crisis

Risk Area	Person—Risk Factors	Caregivers / Environment Assessment
Risk to environment	Has the person damaged or attempted to damage property in recent past? If yes, what was the nature and extent of damage? Does the person have sufficient mobility and strength to be able to cause damage? Does the patient escalate rapidly and/or unpredictably?	Are caregivers able to recognize the escalation and intervene effectively? Do caregivers feel comfortable about being able to predict and prevent it?

Adapted from Surrey Place Centre, 2011

Slide 33

Components
of a Comprehensive Crisis System

1. Crisis Prevention Services
2. Crisis Telephone Services
3. Mobile Crisis Outreach Services
4. Crisis Residential Service
5. Cross-Systems Collaboration

Adapted from Dept of Health & Human Services, nd

Slide 34

**Components
of a Comprehensive Crisis System**

1. Crisis Prevention Services
    a) Proactive, comprehensive, individualized
    b) Designed to avoid a crisis
    c) Accomplished through consultation and education
        - Trained staff
        - Skilled staff
        - Competent staff
    d) Through the development of a crisis prevention plan

Adapted from Dept of Health & Human Services, nd

Slide 35

**Components
of a Comprehensive Crisis System**

2. Crisis Telephone Services
    a) Often the first point of contact
        - Initial triage point
        - Able to reach a wide geographical area
        - Accessible 24 hours a day
    b) Services provided include
        - Supportive communication
        - Consultation
        - Problem-solving
        - Information and referral

Adapted from Dept of Health & Human Services, nd

Slide 36

**Components
of a Comprehensive Crisis System**

3. Mobile Crisis Outreach Services
    a) Provided where the crisis occurs
        - Most feasible
    b) Outreach could occur at
        - Home
        - Work
        - Group home
        - Day services
        - Anywhere in the community

Adapted from Dept of Health & Human Services, nd

M
O
D
U
L
E

8

Slide 37

**Components
of a Comprehensive Crisis System**

4. Crisis Residential Service
    a) Very short-term, highly supervised and supportive residential setting
        • Staffing 24 hours a day
        • Crisis stabilization
        • Trained staff
        • Crisis planning
        • Monitor medications, if needed
        • Linkages to community resources

Adapted from Dept of Health & Human Services, nd

Slide 38

**M
O
D
U
L
E

8**

**Components
of a Comprehensive Crisis System**

4. Crisis Residential Service
    b) Crisis residential settings are:
        • Less restrictive
        • Less disruptive
        • Less costly compared to inpatient programs

Adapted from Dept of Health & Human Services, nd

Slide 39

**Components
of a Comprehensive Crisis System**

5. Cross-Systems Collaboration
    a) Establishment of collaboration among key systems and stakeholders
        • IDD system
        • MH system
        • Education system
        • Forensic system

Adapted from Dept of Health & Human Services, nd

Slide 40

**Components
of a Comprehensive Crisis System**

5.   Cross-Systems Collaboration (cont.)

b)   Collaboration is based on the idea that:

- Negative outcomes result from faulty systems, rather than ineffective people

c)   A dual diagnosis task force:

- Review high-risk individuals
- Make recommendations

Adapted from Dept of Health & Human Services, nd

M
O
D
U
L
E

8

Post-test

Module VIII: Crisis Prevention and Intervention: Reducing Risk

_____ 1. _____ refers to strategies and responses used once signs of crisis are already present.
(a) Behavior modification
(b) Crisis intervention
(c) Crisis prevention
(d) Informed consent

_____ 2. True or false: Most crises can be prevented or interrupted before harm occurs.

_____ 3. A crisis plan should:
(a) Outline what constitutes a crisis for the person and which actions to take to prevent and respond to crises
(b) Include a list of PRN medications to keep administering until the person is calm
(c) Only be used if 911 or other emergency services are called
(d) Require authorization from a psychiatrist

_____ 4. _____ are lifestyle measures (such as relationships, routine and wellness) that minimize the impact of a crisis or prevent a behavior from escalating.
(a) Symptoms
(b) Protective factors
(c) Risk factors
(d) Triggers

_____ 5. Factors that can precipitate a crisis include:
(a) Grief and loss
(b) Medication changes or side effects
(c) Unemployment
(d) All of the above
(e) Only (a) and (b)

_____ 6. Crises can be prevented:
(a) By keeping people isolated from the community and each other
(b) After the first time a person goes to the emergency department
(c) By addressing environmental, biological, psychological and social factors that contribute to behavior
(d) With enough medication

_____ 7. What are some challenges with the current crisis system for people with IDD?
(a) There is a lack of psychiatric services for both adults and children with IDD
(b) Lack of available community programs leads to overutilization of emergency resources
(c) People with IDD are at risk of losing homes or jobs following inpatient admission
(d) All of the above

_____ 8. True or false: Risk assessment used to evaluate a crisis for the general population is not an applicable tool for people with IDD.

_____ 9. During the _____ phase of crisis intervention, helpful responses include supportive verbal techniques, maintaining safety, providing distraction and validation.
(a) Baseline
(b) Prevention
(c) Escalation
(d) Resolution

_____ 10. _____ is based on the idea that negative outcomes result from faulty systems, rather than ineffective people.
(a) Collaboration
(b) Triage
(c) Training
(d) Inclusion

M
O
D
U
L
E

8

Supplemental Materials

Module VIII: Crisis Prevention and Intervention: Reducing Risk

Risk Factors

A crisis is defined as a situation when support needs for a person are greater than what the setting can offer. What are some situations or events that are risk factors for a crisis for a person with IDD/MI?

Consider:
- Think of a person you know with disabilities and mental health needs.

- Reflect on the risk factors you identified above.

- How can we prepare for their changing needs?

_____

_____

Protective Factors

Lifestyle measures can also help prevent a behavior health crisis from escalating. Think of an example of a protective factor in each of the areas below for someone you know.

Protective Factors	Example
Relationships	
Awareness of resources and information	
Routine and predictability	
Valued social/community role	
Wellness supports (mental, physical, emotional)	
Coping skills (relaxation, hobbies)	
Stable housing and work	
Consistent support professionals	

"Crisis," by definition, should not be a regular event. Changes in behavior may indicate changes in need.

Review the examples below and consider how to use information to adjust daily support and expectations to **prevent a crisis** when there are signs of increased needs.

1. When Connie gets on the crowded bus to go to work, she will sometimes repeat the same phrases over and over when she is anxious. If someone bumps into her, she can get into verbal or physical altercations. Today, the bus is very crowded, and she yells to the driver, *"Make room, make room, make room."*

_____

_____

2. After Dwight's mom died, the family sold Dwight's home. Sometimes Dwight will take a bus to his old neighborhood, but he gets lost and ends up very far from his group home.

_____

_____

Reflection

What causes stress in your life?

_____

_____

What things are stressful at your job?

_____

_____

MODULE 8

What are good/bad responses?

_____

_____

How can you be more prepared for a "crisis" on the job when you manage your own stress?

- Identify what factors make you vulnerable to stress.

- Look for clues that you are feeling pressured or anxious.

- Be proactive about your stress triggers.

- Make a stress plan.

Response Planning Worksheet		
Name:		Date:
Predicted behavioral/mental health need:		
What happens as a result of the crisis? List all the outcomes (short term, long term, responses).		
What are the possible causes of and risk factors for the crisis?		
Triggers (environmental, behavioral, physiological, health):		
Observable signs of stress/unmet needs:		

Prevention
(Meeting this person's needs, supporting him/her to feel valuable on an ongoing basis)

What are protective factors (relaxation, routine, predictability, relationships)?	When are they compromised?

What may intensify or escalate the crisis?

Response Steps	
Describe the intervention	Who is responsible for this activity?
1.	
2.	
3.	
4.	
5.	

Long-term follow-up: how can we connect this person to additional supports/protective factors?

M
O
D
U
L
E

8

Module IX

Adapting Therapy Practices

Pre-test

Module IX: Adapting Therapy Practices

_____ 1.   Which of the following is not an adaptation to therapy with people with IDD:
(a) Frequency of sessions
(b) Duration of therapy over time
(c) Therapist needs to be supportive
(d) Longer individual session time

_____ 2.   Which of the following therapeutic modules can apply to individuals with IDD:
(a) Group therapy
(b) Support therapy
(c) Dialectical behavior therapy
(d) All of the above

_____ 3.   The therapist can use the following strategies to modify the complexity of therapy:
(a) The use of repetition for the person to internalize the material discussed in therapy
(b) Breaking down interventions into smaller pieces to ensure understanding before moving on to the next topic of discussion
(c) The use of reflection to ensure understanding of the materials discussed
(d) All of the above

_____ 4.   Finish this sentence with the most appropriate response: Group therapy for people with IDD who have experienced trauma _____.
(a) Helps people foster meaningful relationships and establish a sense of trust, and helps decrease feelings of inadequacy and loneliness
(b) Is not beneficial, as people with IDD cannot benefit from insight-oriented group therapy
(c) Adapts a standard, uniform technique and engages significant others in the therapeutic process
(d) All of the above

_____ 5.   Cognitive Behavior Therapy (CBT) is effective in helping improve a person's overall functioning through:
(a) Psychoanalytic psychotherapy
(b) Applied behavior analysis
(c) Supportive therapy
(d) Skill development and more adaptive cognitive appraisals of events that trigger intense responses

_____ 6. Identify the true statement below:
(a) EMDR is a recommended treatment for people with IDD who have experienced trauma
(b) CBT has not yielded positive results among people with IDD
(c) The general underdiagnosis of PTSD among people who have an IDD does not lead to a large portion of those with PTSD never receiving treatment
(d) Positive identity development is not an effective trauma-informed intervention

_____ 7. The reason communication with collaterals as an adaptation is valuable is because of all except the following:
(a) A therapist should not work in isolation, but be part of the holistic treatment/habilitation/care planning team
(b) If the individual is living with natural family, employing a family-systems approach can be incorporated as an adjunct to individual therapy
(c) Other caregivers can provide important collateral information
(d) Therapists can validate the feelings of the client

_____ 8. True or false: The therapist should never communicate with collaterals.

_____ 9. Guiding principles for instilling hope include the following except:
(a) Using positive language
(b) Staying focused on strengths
(c) Not raising expectations
(d) Celebrating accomplishments

_____ 10. Complete the question with the most appropriate response: A person with IDD may seek therapy _____.
(a) For reasons as varied as the reasons people without IDD seek therapy
(b) People with IDD do not have the same problems as people without IDD
(c) When they have memory retention and self-awareness to participate in traditional models of therapy
(d) Only when their support staff have thoroughly assessed the nature of their maladaptive behavior

Slide 1

Module IX

Adapting Therapy Practices

Slide 2

This module introduces concepts in adapting therapy to make it more useful for persons with IDD.

Slide 3

Learning Objectives

- List therapy guidelines
- Describe ways to adapt psychotherapy practices
- Describe therapeutic models

MODULE 9

Slide 4

Myths About Psychotherapy

Myth: Persons with IDD are not appropriate for psychotherapy.

Premise: Impairments in cognitive abilities and language skills make psychotherapy ineffective.

Reality: Level of intelligence is not a sole indicator for appropriateness of therapy.

Treatment Applications: Psychotherapy approaches need to be adapted to the expressive and receptive language skills of the person.

Fletcher et al. 2015

Slide 5

Facts

- Individuals with ID are at high risk for mental health problems (Summers, Fletcher & Bradley, 2017).
- Significant mental health problems occur in 30-50 percent of people with ID (Fletcher et al., 2016).
- In recent years, research on psychotherapy with persons with ID has advanced (Prout, Brooke, Browning, 2011).
- There is a burgeoning acceptance of the efficacy of psychotherapy with persons with ID and the adaptations that are needed (Shankland & Dagnan, 2015).

Slide 6

Definition of Psychotherapy

- Relationship between a client and a therapist/counselor

- Engaged in a therapeutic relationship

- To achieve a change in emotions, thoughts or behavior

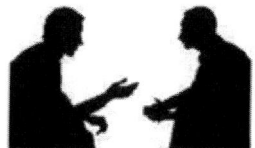

Slide 7

Adapted Therapies

Many typical therapy sessions start with this question: "Have you been feeling better since last time I saw you?"

- Must remember feelings from last visit
- Must know current feelings
- Must be able to compare
- Must know what the therapist is really asking

And so on and so on...

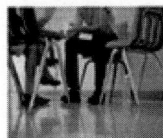

Slide 8

Helping People Cope with Their Daily Problems
A Problem-Solving Model

Slide 9

Why Do People with IDD Need Therapy?

- People with IDD often experience difficulties in coping with daily problems.
- People with IDD have a history of being devalued, leading to feelings of defeat and inadequacy.
- Coping requires self-awareness and a plan for coping in challenging situations.
- People with IDD experience a host of bio-psycho-social vulnerabilities.

Slide 10

**Challenges When Helping
People with IDD**

- Limitations in expressive and receptive language
- Difficulty understanding abstractions
- Difficulty connecting cause and effect
- Poor self-concept

Slide 11

Present Problem

- What is the immediate behavior?
- Is the person anxious or angry?
- How can the therapist help individuals to feel supported so they can better cope with the problem?

Slide 12

Help People Better Cope with Problems

1. Listen
2. Reflect
3. Probe
4. Support
5. Facilitate problem-solving
6. Evaluate outcome

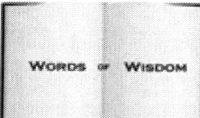

WORDS OF WISDOM

YAI

Slide 13

Therapy Model

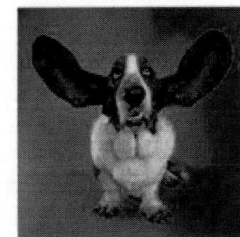

Active Listening

- Attentive
- Interested

Slide 14

Exercise

Pair up and practice active listening. Each person gets to be the client and the listener. Make sure to use the active listening strategies described on the previous slides.

Slide 15

Therapy Model

Reflect

- Repeat a few words.
- Reflection demonstrates active listening.

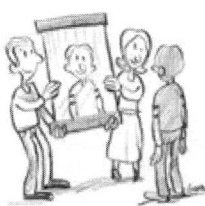

Slide 16

Therapy Model

Probe

- Ask direct questions.
- Avoid interrogation.
- *How* and *what* questions are usually easier to answer than *why* questions.

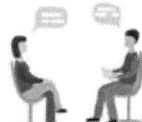

Slide 17

Therapy Model

Support

- Supportive statements indicate understanding.
- Express that you care.
- Acknowledge having been in a similar situation.

Slide 18

Therapy Model

Facilitate problem-solving

- Explore alternative options.
- Support acceptable solutions.

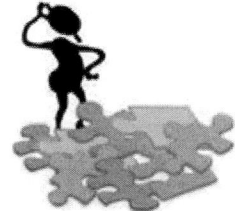

MODULE 9

Slide 19

Therapy Model

Evaluate Outcome

- Was the outcome acceptable?

- Was it positive?

- What was learned?

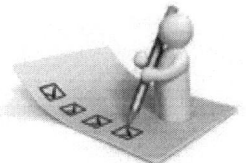

Fletcher, 2007

Slide 20

Encouraging Hope: Guiding Principles

- Use language that promotes hope.

- Raise expectations of what people are capable of accomplishing.

- Stay focused on strengths.

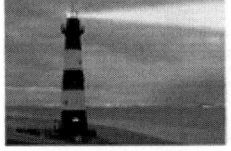

Slide 21

Encouraging Hope: Guiding Principles

- Build everyone's hope.

- Instill a source of hope whenever possible.

- Feeling a sense of hope for the future can be transformative.

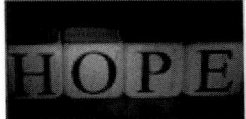

Slide 22

Encouraging Hope: Guiding Principles

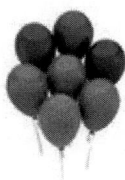

- Celebrate accomplishments.
- Find ways to listen to the people you serve.

Slide 23

Clinician Characteristics

Warmth: Ability to be encouraging and offer positive reinforcement where appropriate while utilizing an empathic approach coupled with an informal and friendly attitude toward the individual. This improves response and motivation to engage in therapy.

Genuineness: Being honest without being too harsh or judgmental. Avoid the misinterpretation of directness as criticism, hostility or rejection.

Ability to develop rapport: Fostering security and trust to counter possible previous experiences of distorted ideas and representations of therapists or authority figures in general. Overcoming this hurdle is essential to effective treatment.

Fletcher et al., 2011

Slide 24

Therapy Guidelines

Intellectual disability affects many aspects of the person's day-to-day life.

People with an intellectual disability usually have some difficulty:
- communicating
- remembering things
- understanding social rules
- understanding cause and effect for everyday events
- solving problems and thinking logically
- reacting and interacting in ways that are characteristic for their age

Fletcher et al., 2011

MODULE 9

Slide 25

Therapy Guidelines

- Use appropriate language
- Speak clearly and slowly.
- Speak in a calm, quiet voice.
- Use simple, short statements or questions.
- Avoid using abstract ideas and jargon.
- Be specific.
- Use a normal tone; don't shout or raise your voice.
- Use non-threatening language (including body language).

Fletcher et al., 2011

Slide 26

Therapy Guidelines

- **Ask one question or make one request at a time.** Keep the conversation simple.

- **Avoid using leading questions.** People with intellectual disability are often suggestible and will tell you what they think you want to hear or what they think is the "right" answer.

- **Use open questions** where possible, e.g., "How are you feeling?" or "Tell me about ...." Closed questions may be useful to clarify something; however, be careful they are not leading questions.

Morasky (2007)

Slide 27

Therapy Guidelines

- **Check the person's understanding from time to time.** If you are not sure they have understood, ask them to explain to you in their own words what you have just asked or said.
- **Do not assume** the person's ability to express themselves is an indication of how much they understand.
- **Be patient**; give the person time to respond.
- **Don't assume** the person with an intellectual disability is able to generalize skills learned in one context or situation automatically to another.
- **Don't pretend to understand.** Use checking questions or paraphrasing to assist your understanding. Ask them to repeat what they have said in another way if they can.

Morasky, 2007

Slide 28

Therapy Guidelines

- Ensure the privacy of the person within the boundaries of confidentiality.
- Be prepared to repeat information more than once if necessary.
- Listen to the person. Don't be judgmental, critical or sarcastic in your response.
- Appear calm, relaxed and confident and provide respect and dignity.
- Keep an upbeat attitude, reassure the person and let them know you are available and supportive.
- Do not make any promises that cannot be kept.
- If the person is alone, ask whether they want family or a support professional involved in therapy. They may have contact details on them.

Morasky, 2007

Slide 29

Multimodal Assessment Considerations

- Medical history
- Medication history
- Developmental history
- Etiology and type of developmental disability
- Trauma/abuse history
- Known problems in other family members
- Forensic history
- Ability level
- Residential history
- Educational history
- Vocational history
- Communication style and ability
- Substance use history

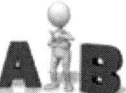

DM-ID 2

Slide 30

Multimodal Assessment Considerations

- Recent life changes
- Changes in vegetative functioning
- Changes in motor functioning
- Changes in cognitive functioning
- Changes in identity/orientation
- Behavioral concerns/changes
- Changes in mood
- Concerns regarding substance abuse

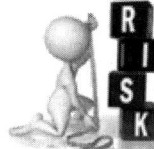

DM-ID 2

Slide 31

Therapeutic Principles

- Empathetic understanding
- Respect and acceptance of people we support
- Concreteness
- Confidentiality
- Draw the person out
- Express genuine interest
- Be aware of your own feelings

Fletcher, et al. (Eds.), 2015

Slide 32

Confidentiality

- Nothing discussed in therapy will be released without the person's permission.

- With the client's permission, the therapist will work collaboratively other care providers.

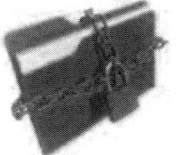

Fletcher, et al. (Eds), 2015

Slide 33

Cognitive Load of Therapy and Intervention

Cognitive load refers to the amount of information and interactions processed simultaneously (or) thinking and reasoning required for people to build on what they already understand.

- Many of the typical ways we provide therapy are complex and require significant cognitive functioning to work.
- Typical practices may not work for a person with IDD.

MODULE 9

Slide 34

Cognitive Processes

- Typical therapy might require inductive reasoning.
  - Therapists help see patterns across multiple incidents.
  - This requires a person to make connections from multiple examples.
- Typical therapy might require deductive reasoning.
  - Therapists help to figure out how to handle certain situations using general rules.
- Typical therapy might require self-awareness to report on feelings and insights about actions and situations.
- These can be difficult for a person with IDD.

Baker, 2011

Slide 35

Ten Adaptations of Therapy

1. Language
2. Frequency of sessions
3. Shorter sessions
4. Duration of therapy
5. Utilize a more structured and directive approach
6. Communication with collaterals
7. Modify complexity of interventions
8. Therapist needs to be supportive
9. Therapist needs to be flexible
10. Use of visual supports

Slide 36

Adaptations of Therapy

1) Language

- Need to understand person's level of language skills
- Need to know the expressive and receptive language skills of the person
- Need to adjust the language used by the therapist that correlates with the language skills of the client
- Adapted to person's cognitive level

Anderson & Kazantzis, 2008

MODULE 9

239

Slide 37

Adaptations of Therapy

2) **Frequency of Sessions**
   - In the beginning stage of therapy, it may be useful to have sessions held more frequently than one would with a neurotypical person.
   - It takes more time to establish a therapeutic relationship as compared to a neurotypical person.
   - For some people, it may be recommended to have therapy two times per week for a relatively brief period of time, and then weekly.

Fletcher et al. (Eds.), 2015

Slide 38

Adaptations of Therapy

3) **Shorter Sessions**
   - There may be a challenge to maintain the person's attention and focus on therapeutic issues that last the usual 45-60 minutes.
   - Allow for a degree of flexibility with regard to the length of any given therapy session.
   - For some people, a 30-minute session is the time period for which their cognitive reserve will allow them the maximum benefit.

Fletcher et al. (Eds.), 2015

Slide 39

Adaptations of Therapy

4) **Duration of Therapy**
   - Increase length of treatment to allow for needed repetition.
   - Increase length of treatment to allow for newly acquired skill sets to be generalized.
   - Increase length of treatment to build upon therapeutic relationship and needed time to work on goals and objectives.
   - Effective termination process may take longer.

Fletcher et al. (Eds.), 2015

MODULE 9

Slide 40

Adaptations of Therapy

5) Utilize a More Structured and Directive Approach

- Structure is often needed in therapy to help bring and maintain focus on the therapeutic material being addressed.
- A more directive approach can be useful to facilitate meaningful interaction between the therapist and the person.
- Silence can be perceived as rejection.

Fletcher et al. (Eds.), 2015

Slide 41

Adaptations of Therapy

6) Communication with Other Care Providers

- With appropriate permission, therapist should communicate with others (care providers, parents, psychiatrist, residential staff, etc.).
- Therapist should not work in isolation, but be part of the holistic treatment/habilitation/care planning team.
- If individual is living with natural family, employing a family systems approach can be incorporated as an adjunct to individual therapy.
- Other caregivers can provide important collateral information.

Fletcher et al. (Eds.), 2015

Slide 42

Adaptations of Therapy

7) Modify complexity of interventions to be in sync with the person's developmental framework

- Repetition is important in order for the person to internalize the material discussed in therapy.
- Discuss one therapeutic issue at a time with attention to beginning, middle and end stages of the material discussed.
- Break down interventions into smaller pieces to ensure understanding before moving on to the next topic of discussion.
- Use reflection to ensure understanding the materials discussed.

Fletcher et al. (Eds.), 2015

M
O
D
U
L
E

9

Slide 43

Adaptations of Therapy

8) **The therapist needs to be supportive**
- Provide a lot of support.
- Give recognition to even small improvements.
- Provide a sense of hope.

Fletcher et al. (Eds.), 2015

Slide 44

Adaptations of Therapy

9) **The therapist needs to be flexible**
- For neurotypical people, when progress is not made, the therapist might assume resistance. With people who have IDD, the therapist needs to adjust and consider an alternative approach.
- An elective approach or at least the knowledge and skills of using more than one model is suggested.
- A supportive approach can be beneficial.

Fletcher et al. (Eds.), 2015

Slide 45

Adaptations of Therapy

10) **Use of visual supports**

Employing visual supports, such as graphics and pictures, can help a person increase their understanding of the therapeutic process:
- Flip charts
- Games
- Social stories
- Handouts
- Multisensory approach

Fletcher et al. (Eds.), 2015

Slide 46

Theoretical Orientation

Just as with the general population, people with intellectual disability and co-occurring mental illness respond to a variety of therapeutic approaches.

A clinician's approach should be informed based on the need of the identified person, rooted in sound, evidence-based theory and supported by education, experience and exposure, relative to providing the treatment.

Fletcher et al. (Eds.), 2015

Slide 47

Therapy Techniques Can Be Adapted

- Cognitive Behavior Therapy (CBT)
- Dialectical Behavior Therapy (DBT)
- Trauma Focused (TF-CBT)
- Group Therapy (GT)
- Support Therapy (SP)
- Other approaches that can be modified
    - Interactive Behavioral Treatment (IBT)
    - Eye Movement Desensitization and Reprocessing (EMDR)
    - Positive psychology

Fletcher et al., 2011

Slide 48

Cognitive Behavior Therapy (CBT)

- CBT is evidenced-based practice
- Based on theory that faulty thinking patterns and beliefs cause both maladaptive behavior and negative emotions
  Targets:
    - Faulty thinking patterns
    - Maladaptive behaviors

- CBT is designed to help client identify and change:
    - Dysfunctional thinking
    - Behavior
    - Emotional responses

Jackson & Gentile, 2011

Slide 49

Characteristics of CBT

1. Thoughts cause feelings and behaviors
2. Time limited to between 16-30 sessions, approximately
3. Emphasis placed on current behavior
4. Teaches the benefits of remaining calm or neutral when faced with difficult situations:

    If you are upset by a problem, then you have two problems:
    - The problem
    - Your upsetness

Jackson & Gentile, 2011

Slide 50

Characteristics of CBT (cont.)

5. Based on relational thought
6. It is structured and directive, based on the notion that maladaptive behaviors are the result of skill deficits.
7. Based on the assumption that most emotional and behavioral reactions are learned; need to unlearn and find new ways of reacting.

Jackson & Gentile, 2011

Slide 51

Cognitive Behavior Therapy

CBT is effective in helping clients improve functioning and in identifying the beliefs, feelings and behaviors associated with the trauma responses.

Overall functioning is improved through skills development and more adaptive cognitive appraisals of events that trigger intense responses.

CBT teaches people to monitor thoughts and change thought patterns that lead to problems. There is a strong evidence base showing utility for persons with IDD if proper adaptation is made (Gaus, 2007).

Jackson & Gentile, 2011

MODULE 9

Slide 52

Trauma-Focused Cognitive Behavioral Therapy

- People are provided knowledge and skills related to processing the trauma; managing distressing thoughts, feelings and behaviors; and enhancing safety.
- TFCBT combines trauma and sensitive interventions with DBT.

Slide 53

Adaptations of CBT for persons with IDD

- Increase the number of sessions to help the person understand abstract concepts.
- Use repetition to help the person with internalization of the material under discussion.
- Involve care providers to assist the person in identifying cognitive distortions.
- Enlist care providers to assist with homework assignments.

Jackson & Gentile, 2011

Slide 54

Dialectical Behavior Therapy (DBT)

- Established by Marsha Linehan (1993).
- DBT is an evidenced-based practice.
- DBT is a structured, skill-based approached.
- The efficacy of DBT is improved when the focus is on building replacement skills rather than merely attempting to eliminate problematic behaviors.

Linehan, 1993

Slide 55

Dialectical Behavior Therapy

DBT is a type of CBT and focuses on helping people:

- Learn to regulate their emotions
- Improve ability to cope with stress

DBT comprises two main components:

1. Weekly individual sessions
2. Weekly group sessions

Linehan, 1993

Slide 56

Dialectical Behavior Therapy

DBT is a comprehensive treatment program addressing deficits in emotion regulation, distress tolerance and interpersonal relationships accomplished through:

- individual psychotherapy
- skills training groups
- supervision/case consultation groups

Linehan, 1993

Slide 57

Adaptations of DBT for Persons with IDD

- Principles of treatment remain the same, but the presentation and language are modified
- Concepts are pared down or simplified
- Handouts are rewritten to increase attention and aid in understanding
- Much individual feedback is provided
- Repetition is used to assist with learning, retention and generalization
- Shorter time for individual and group treatment

Charlton & Dykstra, 2011

Slide 58

Group Therapy

- Group Therapy (GT) affords the opportunity to address problems with the support of others who may have common issues and goals.
- The result is a sense of universality as clients realize that others share similar struggles.
- GT can be process-oriented, and there is benefit in witnessing the resourcefulness of the group members who are in a similar situation.

Fletcher & Duffy, 1993

Slide 59

Group Therapy

- Group members can gain a sense of reassurance and hope in their own recovery
- GT provides a safe environment to experience validation and normalcy
- GT benefits include
  - Improved interpersonal relationships
  - Improved problem-solving skills
  - Improved acceptance of self, leading to improved self-esteem and acceptance

Fletcher & Duffy 1993

Slide 60

Interactive Behavioral Treatment (IBT)

A group therapy treatment for trauma that uses person-to-person interaction, psychodrama and therapeutic interventions as an interactive method to address trauma and related conditions.

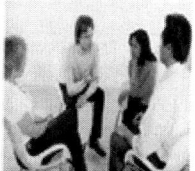

Razza & Tomasulo (2005).

Slide 61

Supportive Psychotherapy (SP)

- Supportive therapy (SP) incorporates a variety of therapy theories.
- It is interactive between therapist and client.
- SP is based on the belief that a supportive relationship can serve to help the client make a positive change.
- Therapist assumes a strong empathetic stance and nurturing positive transference, which strengthens the relationship.

Jackson & Gentile, 2012

Slide 62

Supportive Psychotherapy (SP)

- SP primarily focuses on "here and now" issues.
- Therapist facilitates improved affect regulation, improved healthy emotional response to stress and improved interpersonal relationships.
- Modification with people who have IDD
  - Reduce complexity by shrinking down time into smaller units
  - Augment with games, drawings, role play, etc.
  - Therapy may involve family and/or others who have significant impact on the client.

Jackson & Gentile, 2012

Slide 63

Eye Movement Desensitization and Reprocessing (EMDR)

- First developed by Francine Shapiro upon noticing that certain eye movements reduced the intensity of disturbing thought.
- EMDR uses a person's own rapid, rhythmic eye movements.
- Treatment consists of eight phases with precise intentions.

Shapiro, 2012

Slide 64

Positive Psychology for People with ID/MI

There has been a recent shift in the conceptualization of intellectual disability, with increased attention directed toward the importance of identifying and enhancing the strengths and capabilities of people with intellectual disabilities as a means to promote meaningful participation, community inclusion and quality-of-life outcomes.

Positive psychological approach seeks to increase human flourishing and optimal functioning. For people with ID and MI, their strengths and virtues are recognized and developed to enable them to thrive.

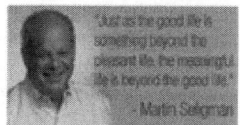

"Just as the good life is something beyond the pleasant life, the meaningful life is beyond the good life."
– Martin Seligman

Shogren, Wehmeyer & Singh (Eds.), 2017

Slide 65

Summary

By adapting empirically validated psychotherapy techniques and treatments, a clinician can provide effective therapy for people with IDD/MI.

With some consideration to cognitive abilities, including expressive and receptive language, psychotherapy techniques can be effectively adapted to meet the needs of people who have IDD/MI.

Post-test

Module IX: Adapting Therapy Practices

_____ 1.   Which of the following is not an adaptation to therapy with people with IDD:
(a) Frequency of sessions
(b) Duration of therapy over time
(c) Therapist needs to be supportive
(d) Longer individual session time

_____ 2.   Which of the following therapeutic modules can apply to individuals with IDD:
(a) Group therapy
(b) Support therapy
(c) Dialectical behavior therapy
(d) All of the above

_____ 3.   The therapist can use the following strategies to modify the complexity of therapy:
(a) The use of repetition for the person to internalize the material discussed in therapy
(b) Breaking down interventions into smaller pieces to ensure understanding before moving on to the next topic of discussion
(c) The use of reflection to ensure understanding of the materials discussed
(d) All of the above

_____ 4.   Finish this sentence with the most appropriate response: Group therapy for people with IDD who have experienced trauma _____ .
(a) Helps people foster meaningful relationships and establish a sense of trust, and helps decrease feelings of inadequacy and loneliness
(b) Is not beneficial, as people with IDD cannot benefit from insight-oriented group therapy
(c) Adapts a standard, uniform technique and engages significant others in the therapeutic process
(d) All of the above

_____ 5.   Cognitive Behavior Therapy (CBT) is effective in helping improve a person's overall functioning through:
(a) Psychoanalytic psychotherapy
(b) Applied behavior analysis
(c) Supportive therapy
(d) Skill development and more adaptive cognitive appraisals of events that trigger intense responses

_____ 6. Identify the true statement below:
(a) EMDR is a recommended treatment for people with IDD who have experienced trauma
(b) CBT has not yielded positive results among people with IDD
(c) The general underdiagnosis of PTSD among people who have an IDD does not lead to a large portion of those with PTSD never receiving treatment
(d) Positive identity development is not an effective trauma-informed intervention

_____ 7. The reason communication with collaterals as an adaptation is valuable is because of all except the following:
(a) A therapist should not work in isolation, but be part of the holistic treatment/ habilitation/care planning team
(b) If the individual is living with natural family, employing a family-systems approach can be incorporated as an adjunct to individual therapy
(c) Other caregivers can provide important collateral information
(d) Therapists can validate the feelings of the client

_____ 8. True or false: The therapist should never communicate with collaterals.

_____ 9. Guiding principles for instilling hope include the following except:
(a) Using positive language
(b) Staying focused on strengths
(c) Not raising expectations
(d) Celebrating accomplishments

_____ 10. Complete the question with the most appropriate response: A person with IDD may seek therapy _____.
(a) For reasons as varied as the reasons people without IDD seek therapy
(b) People with IDD do not have the same problems as people without IDD
(c) When they have memory retention and self-awareness to participate in traditional models of therapy
(d) Only when their support staff have thoroughly assessed the nature of their maladaptive behavior

Supplemental Materials

Module IX: Adapting Therapy Practices

Historical Reasons for Lack of Psychotherapy

- Myth that problem behaviors are part of IDD (diagnostic overshadowing)

- Not viewed as effective due to lower IQ

- Mental health provider's negative bias

- Near absence of professional training

Exercise

Why is psychotherapy with people who have IDD more accepted now as compared to the past?

_____

_____

Adaptations — Flexibility

Many typical therapy sessions start with this question: "How have you been feeling since our last session?" This may not be appropriate because of these reasons:

- Must be able to remember feelings from last session

- Must be cognizant of current feelings

- Must be able to inductively reason

Exercise

What are some other ways to start a session?

_____

_____

M
O
D
U
L
E

9

Implications for Group Therapy

There are numerous therapeutic effects of group therapy. Here are a few:

- Fosters relationships

- Enables learning through participation

- Promotes sense of belonging

- Promotes peer support and group cohesion

- Helps decrease feelings of isolation and failure

Exercise

Can you name other benefits of group therapy?

M
O
D
U
L
E

9

Case Vignette

Amy is a 25-year-old female with a mild level of ID and a diagnosis of bipolar disorder. She lives with her mother in a suburban neighborhood. Amy is in a supportive work environment five days a week and reportedly is doing well. Recently she has reported in therapy feelings of anger and resentment, especially toward her mother. She reports that she wants to be more independent. This has caused a strain on the relationship between mother and daughter, and they have been having frequent arguments.

Exercise

If you are the therapist in this case scenario, what treatment techniques or strategies would you employ?

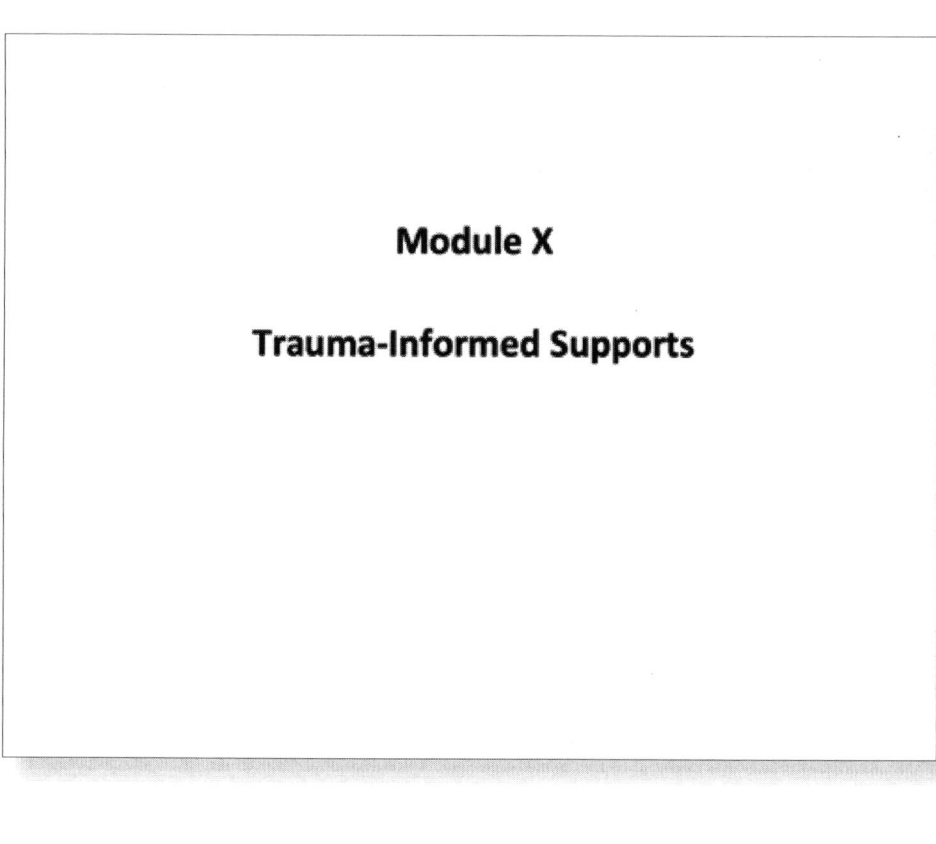

Module X

Trauma-Informed Supports

Pre-test

Module X: Trauma-Informed Supports

_____ 1. When Xavier was a teenager, he was abused by a staff member at his school program. He is afraid of men who wear neckties and eyeglasses. What is a trauma-informed intervention to support Xavier?
(a) Limit his DSPs and social relationships to women only
(b) Identify what makes Xavier feel safe and provide it when he encounters a trigger
(c) Take him to places and events where only family members are present
(d) Give Xavier a PRN of an antianxiety medication when he goes out

_____ 2. _____ trauma refers to the type of trauma experienced by hearing about abuse or encounters that happened to other people.
(a) Vicarious
(b) Direct
(c) Complex
(d) Chronic

_____ 3. Whether or not trauma leads to longer-term issues, such as a disorder, depends on:
(a) The type of developmental disability a person has
(b) Duration, intensity and intentionality of trauma
(c) Whether the person has verbal language
(d) If the person takes medication following the event

_____ 4. Possible trauma events for individuals with IDD include:
(a) Uncertainty of safety and basic needs being met
(b) Witnessing violence
(c) Loss of home or job or support services
(d) All of the above

_____ 5. True or false: Everyone will be exposed to events in their lifetime that put them at risk of post-traumatic stress disorder.

_____ 6. _____ means understanding how trauma affects a person and knowing effective strategies to help them achieve safety and wellness
(a) Trauma-informed
(b) Avoidance behavior
(c) "Fight or flight"
(d) Positive identity development

MODULE 10

_____ 7. Trauma is processed and stored in the _____ system of the body
   (a) Nervous
   (b) Circulatory
   (c) Limbic
   (d) Digestive

_____ 8. Three keys to recovery in a trauma-informed support are:
   (a) Therapy, medication and behavior modification
   (b) Safety, connection and empowerment
   (c) Redirection, refocusing and reframing
   (d) Compliance, consequences and counseling

_____ 9. Behaviors that may stem from a history of trauma include:
   (a) Eating nonedible items
   (b) Entering others' personal space
   (c) Refusing medications
   (d) All of the above

_____ 10. True or false: Once a person's identity is established, it cannot be improved or changed.

MODULE 10

Slide 1

Module X

Trauma-Informed Supports

Slide 2

Learning Objectives

Participants will

- Identify risks of individuals with IDD for developing trauma-related disorders.
- Recognize how trauma history can present as challenging behavior.
- Identify methods for adapting trauma treatment and supports for individuals with IDD.

Slide 3

Trauma

- Trauma is the emotional response to a terrible event like an accident, rape or natural disaster.
- Immediately after the event, shock and denial are typical.
- Longer-term reactions include unpredictable emotions, flashbacks, strained relationships and even physical symptoms, such as headaches or nausea (APA, 2013).

M
O
D
U
L
E

1
0

Slide 4

A major trauma could be:

- Sexual assault/physical assault
- Natural or manmade disasters
- Catastrophic illness
- Loss of a loved one
- Humiliation
- Bullying
- Deprivation and powerlessness to act on one's own behalf

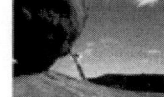

Palay, 2012

Slide 5

Types of Trauma

- **Single or event** — occurs one time (car accident, one instance of abuse, witnessing a death).
- **Complex** (in contrast to single) — over time, prolonged (repeated abuse, target of bullying, moving frequently, living in a situation of continuous conflict).
- **Direct** — death of a loved one, car accident, illness.
- **Vicarious** (in contrast to direct) — through experience of others (hearing about abuse from a friend, being a therapist listening to others' experiences, child or abused parent).

Slide 6

Simple and Complex PTSD

"Big T" Traumas
Simple post-traumatic stress results from a one-time incident, such as a rape, violent assault or injury.

"Little t" Traumas
Complex post-traumatic stress is a complex set of responses that follows chronic, multiple and/or ongoing traumatic events such as taunting, teasing, tormenting or prolonged abuse.

Harvey, 2009

MODULE 10

Slide 7

Possible Trauma Events for Individuals with IDD

- Abuse: verbal, physical, sexual
- Bullying
- Identified as being different
- Being restrained or forced seclusion (re-traumatizing)
- The "R" word, other disparaging language
- Constant threats (perceived or actual)
- Moving away from family, loss, grief
- Uncertainty of safety and basic needs being met
- Witnessing violence
- Loss of home or job or support services
- Add medical and dental problems, costly prescriptions

Slide 8

Levels of Stress:
What Types of Events Cause Trauma?

A Continuum

Normal or "routine" stress

Tolerable but depleting stress

Toxic - Traumatic stress

Slide 9

Trauma

People with intellectual/developmental disabilities are at greater risk for being victimized or abused.

Some experts believe as many as 90 percent of people with intellectual disabilities have some level of traumatic stress. Sobsey (1994) reports that people with disabilities are twice as likely to experience abuse.

Sobsey, 1994

M
O
D
U
L
E

1
0

Slide 10

People with Disabilities Are at Greater Risk of Being Victimized

- More than one in five people from ages 12-19 report sexual violence.
- Three times more likely to experience violent victimization as adolescents and adults.
- Three times more likely to experience rape, sexual assault, aggravated assault and robbery.
- Three times more likely to be sexually abused as children.
- 1.6 times more likely to experience abuse or neglect as children.
- 1.5 times more likely to experience repeated abuse or neglect as children.
- This includes women with disabilities, people with cognitive or developmental disabilities, people with psychiatric illness and people with multiple disabilities.

© 2019 Center on Victimization and Safety
Vera Institute of Justice

Slide 11

Risk Factors

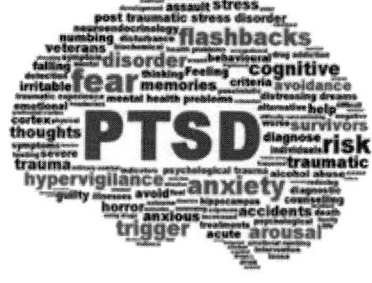

Slide 12

Risk Factors for Developing Trauma Disorders

Risk Factors	Protective Factors
Multiple traumas	Timely and appropriate care
Acquiescence/passivity	Social supports
Lack of control	Safety awareness
Underdeveloped/ineffective coping skills	Previous experience
Communication difficulties	Good communication skills
Mood or anxiety disorder	Wellness supports
Age at time of event	Coping skills
Likely to have less inductive and deductive reasoning	Experiences cognitive dissonance
Isolation and exclusion	Stable housing and work

Slide 13

DSM-5: Trauma- and Stressor-Related Disorders

Include: Reactive Attachment Disorder, Post-traumatic Stress Disorder, Acute Stress Disorder.

PTSD is the most common.
- History of exposure to traumatic events (stressors)
- Presence of intrusion symptoms: reliving trauma, flashbacks
- Avoidance behaviors in effort to escape distress
- Alterations in arousal and reactivity following the trauma (e.g., irritable aggressive behavior or self-destructive behavior)
- Symptoms persist longer than one month after trauma

Trauma brings the past into the present.

Slide 14

People with IDD often manifest PTSD differently than what is typically recognized as PTSD in the DSM–5.

Some individuals may have flashbacks but are not able to communicate that experience. What they do communicate, rather, may be misunderstood as a psychotic disorder.

Slide 15

DM-ID-2 PTSD

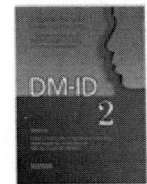

Behaviors

A. Agitation/property destruction
B. Obsessive behavior
C. Paranoia
D. Noncompliance
E. Aggression
F. "Shutdown"
G. Escape behavior

Symptoms

A. Arousal (hyperarousal)
B. Avoidance (hypervigilance)
C. Mistrust based on abuse experiences
D. Dissociation
E. Fight response based on triggering of amygdala and sympathetic nervous system
F. Freeze response
G. Flight response

Slide 16

Trauma and ASD: Symptoms and Diagnosis

Pathology	Trauma symptomology	Autism traits
Impaired stress response	• Sensitivity to traumatic reminders • Alternation in neuroendocrine stress response system	• Sensitivity to traumatic reminders • Alternation in neuroendocrine stress response system
Disturbance in sense of self and identity	• Suicidality • Self-mutilation • Low self-esteem • Risk-taking • Depersonalization	• Self-mutilation • Low self-esteem • Depersonalization
Interpersonal and relationship problems	• Attachment disorders • Social withdrawal • Promiscuity • Antisocial behavior	• Attachment disorders • Social withdrawal • Antisocial behavior
Affect dysregulation	• Use and abuse of substances to regulate mood, sense of self and behavior • Attention problems • ADHD symptoms • Impulsivity • Hypervigilance	• Attention problems • ADHD symptoms • Impulsivity • Hypervigilance

http://www.traumainformedcareproject.org/

Slide 17

Trauma and the Mind

When a trigger/stressor is introduced:

- **Amygdala** activated by stressors, activates release hormones
- **Cortex** processes information
- **Limbic system** activated: fight, flight or freeze
- **Hippocampus** is working memory
  - stores experiences and cause
  - breaks down when there is too much stress
  - interrupts learning and remembering behavioral tasks when overworked

Prolonged stress causes permanent damage due to increased levels of cortisol and adrenaline.

Slide 18

Trauma and the Body

The body stores trauma. The physiological response to threats (real or perceived) takes its toll over time and can manifest as somatic symptoms:

- Gastrointestinal issues
- Exaggerated pain response
- Migraines
- Muscle tension and soreness

MODULE 10

Slide 19

Trauma and Emotions

Emotional states of trauma include anxiety, anger, horror, helplessness and sadness. An individual's experience can fluctuate and include:

- Avoidant behavior, overreaction
- Increased arousal
- Exaggerated startle response, hypervigilance
- Difficulty concentrating
- Outbursts of rage and fear

Slide 20

Behaviors That May Stem from a History of Trauma

- Verbal threats
- Physical aggression
- Running away
- Entering others' personal space
- Refusing medications
- Difficulty sleeping
- Withdrawal
- Hoarding
- Eating quickly
- Eating non-edibles
- Challenges with toileting

Slide 21

Trauma-Informed

Being trauma-informed means understanding how trauma affects a person and knowing effective strategies to help them achieve safety and wellness.

Slide 22

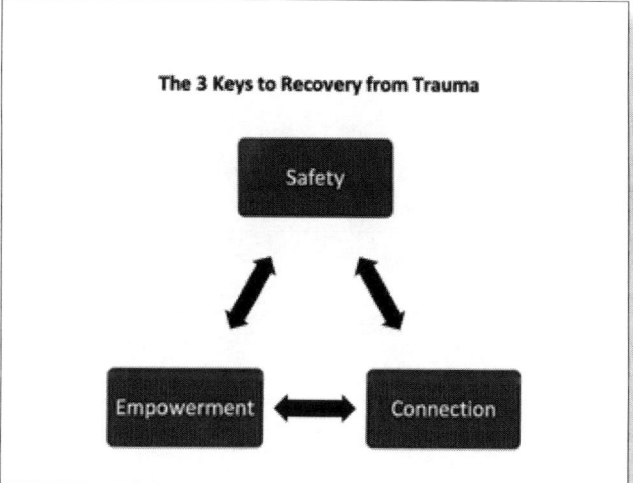

The 3 Keys to Recovery from Trauma

Safety

Empowerment

Connection

Slide 23

Trauma Approach: Safety

People need to feel safe from threats that are real or perceived. This includes:

- Be mindful of behavior that can stem from trauma history
- Introduce relationships slowly
- Creating a structured, predictable, flexible environment
- Be aware of your own body language

Slide 24

Techniques to Help People Feel Safe

- Redirection/Refocusing
- Reframing
  - Change the topic or setting or activity to avoid triggers
- Awareness of your own body language
- Find more supportive and comfortable staff, home, job, neighborhood
- Teach coping skills: breathing, humor, prayer, music

M O D U L E 1 0

Slide 25

Safety: Proactive Supports

Recovery is in not linear. Be mindful and attentive to threats to healing.

- Avoid any kind of re-traumatization from our support strategies (seclusion, isolation, punitive consequences).
- Create a psychiatric advance care directive: Help the person make a plan with steps for support strategies for any setbacks or triggers.

Slide 26

Promote Safe Communication

- Be open to listening
- Show empathy, not judgment
- Be sensitive to the person's triggers
- Use kind words and a calm tone
- Engage in kind actions
- Validate emotions
- Define expectations and roles
- Use visual cues
- Have a predictable staff and activity schedule

Slide 27

Trauma Recovery: Connection

- Include individuals in hiring staff, choosing therapists, other team members.
- Build relationships with trusted people first; expand to new members once rapport is established.
- Create and develop valued roles in the community.
- Support meaningful activities.

M
O
D
U
L
E

1
0

Slide 28

Trauma Recovery: Empowerment

- Provide and honor real choices.
- Support informed decision-making.
- Encourage leadership and organization of others in need of healing support.
- Create and nurture opportunities for self-care, including healthy diet, exercise and sleep.
- Assist in the use of tools and resources.

http://pid.thenadd.org/

Slide 29

Kristina

Kristina is a 24-year-old woman who lives in a group home with two other women. She has anxiety and mild intellectual disability. Kristina is generally a happy and social person. She has a job in a plant nursery watering flowers. When she has free time, she likes to go shopping, go to movies and go out to eat. She does best when her schedule and work are predictable. Kristina tends to stick to activities with which she feels successful.

Kristina has a history of being teased when she was at school, specifically being called names and being told she's *stupid* and *ugly* and excluded from activities. Sometimes at work when a customer asks her a question she can't answer, she will hear her old classmates' voices in her head and run to the breakroom to cry.

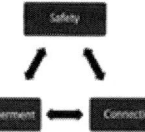

Slide 30

Therapeutic Approaches

- DBT – Dialectical Behavior Therapy
  - Supportive counseling
  - Group therapy
- TF-CBT
- EMDR
- Individual psychotherapy
- Workbook, journaling, guided imagery
- Positive identity development

M
O
D
U
L
E

1
0

Slide 31

Positive Identity Development

Identity is a core construct of self-worth and self-image. Many people with dual diagnosis often see themselves as a person with a disability or disorder. For those with a trauma history, negative experiences or events can disrupt identity. Goals and relationships can be damaged by abuse. Developing a positive identity can be a healing step in recovery.

Slide 32

Positive Identity Development

The presence of an intellectual/developmental disability impacts exposure to new experiences and the person's understanding and integration of those experiences.

This requires the organization and delivery of identity-related supports and counseling for persons with IDD across the life span.

Harvey, 2009

Slide 33

Many people with IDD have a largely negative sense of identity, which is constituted of all the good things the person is not. Specific therapeutic approaches can help to create a more positive sense of identity.

Harvey, 2009

Slide 34

How Is Identity Developed?

- Accumulation of experience
- Learning from experience
- Inductive and deductive reasoning
- Timing
- Attribution of meaning

Steve Dahl, 2019

Slide 35

How Does IDD Affect Identity Development?

- Lower rates of activity, particularly social
- Impeded understanding
- Slower development of logic
- Pattern of compliance and pleasing others – identity foreclosure

Steve Dahl, 2019

Slide 36

Small Group Activity

- Review the factors that contribute to identity development
- How would each be different as a result of having IDD?
- How can this increase trauma risk and impede trauma recovery? (safety, empowerment, connection)

MODULE 10

Slide 37

Resources

Trauma-Informed Project-resources and publications
http://www.traumainformedcareproject.org/resources.php

My Book About Recovery by Karen Harvey (2007)—available free at:
https://aaidd.org/docs/default-source/events/harvey-my-book-about-recovery.pdf?sfvrsn=2

http://pid.thenadd.org/

Trauma and Recovery: The Aftermath of Violence—from Domestic Abuse to Political Terror by Judith Herman, MD (1992)

Behind Closed Doors: The Story of Four Women Struggling to Reconcile Violence within the Psychiatric System (brief documentary):
https://vimeo.com/2709542

Healing Neen (brief documentary): https://vimeo.com/15851924

MODULE 10

Post-test

Module X: Trauma-Informed Supports

_____ 1. When Xavier was a teenager, he was abused by a staff member at his school program. He is afraid of men who wear neckties and eyeglasses. What is a trauma-informed intervention to support Xavier?
(a) Limit his DSPs and social relationships to women only
(b) Identify what makes Xavier feel safe and provide it when he encounters a trigger
(c) Take him to places and events where only family members are present
(d) Give Xavier a PRN of an antianxiety medication when he goes out

_____ 2. _____ trauma refers to the type of trauma experienced by hearing about abuse or encounters that happened to other people.
(a) Vicarious
(b) Direct
(c) Complex
(d) Chronic

_____ 3. Whether or not trauma leads to longer-term issues, such as a disorder, depends on:
(a) The type of developmental disability a person has
(b) Duration, intensity and intentionality of trauma
(c) Whether the person has verbal language
(d) If the person takes medication following the event

_____ 4. Possible trauma events for individuals with IDD include:
(a) Uncertainty of safety and basic needs being met
(b) Witnessing violence
(c) Loss of home or job or support services
(d) All of the above

_____ 5. True or false: Everyone will be exposed to events in their lifetime that put them at risk of post-traumatic stress disorder.

_____ 6. _____ means understanding how trauma affects a person and knowing effective strategies to help them achieve safety and wellness
(a) Trauma-informed
(b) Avoidance behavior
(c) "Fight or flight"
(d) Positive identity development

_____ 7. Trauma is processed and stored in the _____ system of the body
      (a) Nervous
      (b) Circulatory
      (c) Limbic
      (d) Digestive

_____ 8. Three keys to recovery in a trauma-informed support are:
      (a) Therapy, medication and behavior modification
      (b) Safety, connection and empowerment
      (c) Redirection, refocusing and reframing
      (d) Compliance, consequences and counseling

_____ 9. Behaviors that may stem from a history of trauma include:
      (a) Eating nonedible items
      (b) Entering others' personal space
      (c) Refusing medications
      (d) All of the above

_____ 10. True or false: Once a person's identity is established, it cannot be improved or changed.

MODULE 10

Supplemental Materials

Module X: Trauma-Informed Supports

Why do you think people with IDD are more likely (at risk) to experience trauma events?

_____

_____

What are some of these possible trauma events for individuals with IDD?

_____

_____

Below are some examples of protective factors that help people develop resilience when faced with traumatic events. Can you think of an example that applies to someone you know/support with IDD that can help build resilience?

Protective Factors	Example
Social supports (relationships, information)	
Safety awareness	
Previous experience	
Good communication skills	
Wellness supports (mental, physical, emotional)	
Coping skills (relaxation, hobbies)	
Stable housing and work	

MODULE 10

One model to support a trauma-informed approach involves providing Safety, Connection and Empowerment. Safety involves helping the person feel safe from threats that are real or perceived, especially when triggers are present. Connection includes processing the traumatic experience at a safe and manageable pace with someone the person trusts, as well as development of supportive relationships. Empowerment includes development of positive self-identity and making healthy choices.

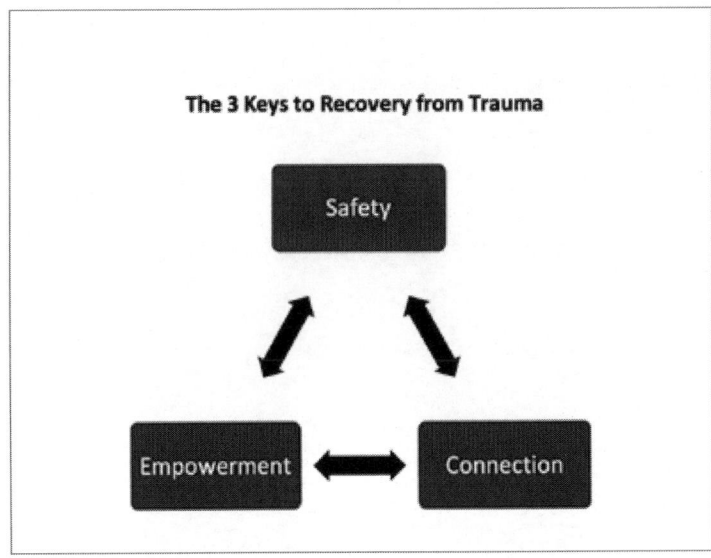

Consider someone you know/support who has been affected by a traumatic experience(s). Using the recovery components of safety, connection and empowerment, how can you support this person to have a better life?

_____

_____

Thinking specifically about safety. What are some techniques you can use to ensure a safe space and conversation with someone? (Hint: Reflect on communication, connection, environment.)

_____

_____

Healing trauma is about restoring and building connections. How can you support yourself or someone you know to build relationships and rapport within your/their circle and community?

_____

_____

M
O
D
U
L
E

1
0

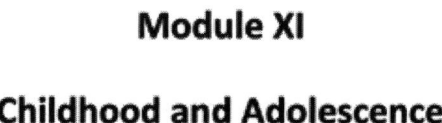

Module XI

Childhood and Adolescence

Pre-test

Module XI: Childhood and Adolescence

_____ 1. Functioning and behavior are influenced by:
(a) The Eltdown gland
(b) Stages of development
(c) A static pathway all young people follow
(d) None of the above

_____ 2. Cultural perspectives of the family must:
(a) Always be taken into account
(b) Sometimes be taken into account
(c) Never be taken into account
(d) Be considered only when they clash with treatment goals

_____ 3. One of the first people to study the development of a personal identity was:
(a) Randolph Carter
(b) Tara Maclay
(c) B.F. Skinner
(d) Erik Erikson

_____ 4. A sense of identity includes:
(a) Gender identity
(b) Sense of purpose
(c) Knowledge of character traits
(d) All of the above

_____ 5. Which of the following is not true about most cases of bullying?
(a) It's done by someone with more power or social support to someone with less power or social support
(b) It often includes the abuser blaming the target for the abuse
(c) It often leads to vengeance spells
(d) In most bullying situations, the target cannot stop the bullying by their own actions

_____ 6. Cyberbullying is:
(a) Becoming less common quickly due to efforts by social media companies
(b) Difficult to prosecute due to the court case Gibbous vs. Pnakotic
(c) Likely to cause real-world problems for targets
(d) Not a big worry because it is all online anyway

_____ 7. Which of the following is not a common adolescent problem?
(a) Senescence
(b) Eating disorders
(c) Depression
(d) Substance abuse

_____ 8. Which of the following is an eating disorder?
(a) Anorexia nervosa
(b) Bulimia
(c) Both (a) and (b)
(d) Neither (a) or (b)

_____ 9. Substance dependence is an extra concern for youth with IDD due to:
(a) Lack of understanding of long-term consequences
(b) Greater access to street drugs than typical youth
(c) Higher risk of physical dependence than typical youth
(d) All of the above

_____ 10. What is the best way to help a young person with IDD be safe in the community?
(a) Use Hazred's decision matrix
(b) Teach the young person who and what can be dangerous
(c) Follow the same routines always, as that builds comfort
(d) Look for the appearance of safety

MODULE 11

M
O
D
U
L
E

1
1

Slide 1

Module XI

Childhood and Adolescence

Slide 2

Childhood and Adolescence

Portions of this module were developed originally
by Phil Smith, Ph.D.
Boggs Center on Developmental Disabilities
Rutgers Robert Wood Johnson Medical School

Slide 3

This module describes issues of typical childhood and adolescence
development and details how they are relevant to youth with IDD.

Slide 4

Learning Objectives

- Describe the stages of typical development for younger children and adolescents
- Describe how disability affects self-image/self-esteem
- Describe the issue around development and support for various challenges of maturation

Slide 5

Issues of Development

- There is a typical pathway or sequence of development in which certain cognitive, social and emotional things are seen in each stage for typical people.
- Functioning and behavior are influenced by stages of development.
- Intellectual/developmental disabilities often change development due to difficulties in learning, different patterns of interaction and lack of typical experiences, but most stages still occur (American Academy of Pediatrics, 2013).

Slide 6

It's All About Family

- Support for youth and adolescents with IDD must always consider the family.
- Support for the child must fit within the family system.
- Cultural perspectives of family must always be taken into account.

Baker, 2013, Baker & Blumberg,2013

M
O
D
U
L
E

1
1

Slide 7

Typical Stages

Approximate ages
- Newborn, ages 0-1 month
- Infant, ages 1 month-1 year
- Toddler, ages 1-3 years
- Preschooler, ages 4-6 years
- School-aged child, ages 6-13 years
- Adolescent, ages 13-20

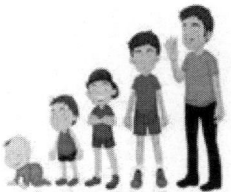

Slide 8

Characteristics of Typical Younger Children

- Often significant issues with attachment and attachment disorders
- Typical developmental tasks related to delaying gratification, task completion and development of a sense of identify
- Many problems related to impulsiveness and lack of empathy

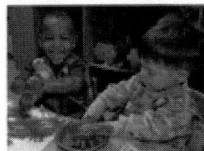

Slide 9

Characteristics of Adolescence

Teen life is complex for all young people, as they ...
- Physically mature
- Sexually mature
- Emotionally mature
  - Desire independence
  - Sense of identity is built
  - Heightened focus on peers
  - Sexual awareness

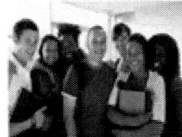

Shelov Remer Altmann, 2009

Slide 10

Adolescence and Disability

An adolescent with an IDD experiences the same life complexities as other adolescents.

The presence of IDD or a physical disability can make learning and making sense of the world more complex.

Slide 11

Self-image, Self-esteem

- Central theme — discovering oneself
  - Creating a personality
  - Shaping a personal image of oneself (very self-conscious)
  - Concerned with outward appearance

- Often focus on the ways they fail to meet the ideal
  - This often results in low self-esteem and unhappiness

- Shapes how they feel peers look at them
- Use what one's peers think to determine their self-image
- Try out roles and test these out through social interaction

Slide 12

Problems with Self-Esteem

Often include:
- Body image
- Weight problems
- Shyness
- Embarrassment

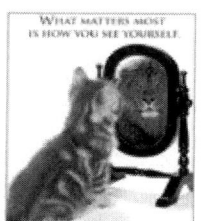

And for someone with IDD, awareness of disability.

Slide 13

Exercise

Please come up with ten words that describe you, ten things that make you who you are.

Slide 14

MODULE 11

Risk-Taking Behavior

- All teenagers take risks as a normal part of growing up.
- Changes in the teen brain make risk-taking more likely.
    - Time of great opportunity
    - Risks and problems as well
- Taking risks is a tool teens use to define and develop their identity.
- Adolescents need to take risks.
    - Healthy risk-taking can help prevent unhealthy risk-taking
    - Help create opportunities for healthy risks

Romer, 2010

Slide 15

Unhealthy Risk-Taking

- Drinking
- Smoking
- Unsafe sex
- Drug use
- Disordered eating
- Stealing
- Gang activity
- Self-mutilation

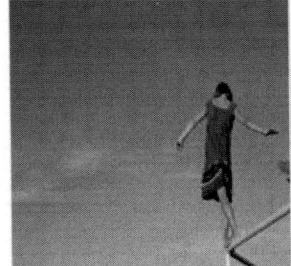

Romer, 2010

Slide 16

Healthy Risk-Taking

- Sports
- Developing artistic abilities
- Volunteer activities
- Travel
- Making new friends
- Hobbies
- Exploring community

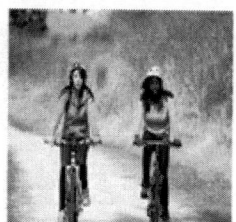

Romer, 2010

Slide 17

Exercise

- Identify two things you do that are examples of healthy risk-taking.

- Then think of one negative risk-taking thing you do, but don't write it down or share it.

Slide 18

Supporting Risk-Taking

All such activities contain the possibility of failure.

- How can we help provide supports that include realistic goals?
- What skills do young people need to make good choices about taking risks?
- What are some challenges unique to younger individuals?

M
O
D
U
L
E

1
1

Slide 19

Sexuality

- Key milestones of adolescent development
  - Attaining an adult body
  - Capable of reproducing
  - Intimate relationships
  - Complex emotions
- Individuals with disabilities may be hindered in this area of development
  - Functional limitations
  - Social isolation
    - Fewer social activities
    - Less likely to have intimate relationships
  - Lack of information on parenthood, birth control and STDs

Watson, Griffiths, Richards & Dykstra, 2002

Slide 20

Development of Sexuality

- Children and adolescents with IDD, like all individuals, are sexual persons.
- Most of their behaviors are "typical."
- The problem is they are often unable to distinguish between behaviors that are publicly and privately appropriate.
- Attention to medical, functional and behavioral issues may shift focus away from addressing sexuality.

Watson, Griffiths, Richards, & Dykstra, 2002

Slide 21

Supports

- Avoid judgment and projection of personal values or discomfort
- Ensure the privacy of each child and adolescent
- Promote self-care and social independence among persons with disabilities
- Advocate for appropriate sexuality education
- Help provide knowledge and/or identify a source of information
- Lack of attention to issues of sexuality can lead to misinformation and problem behavior

Slide 22

Sex Education

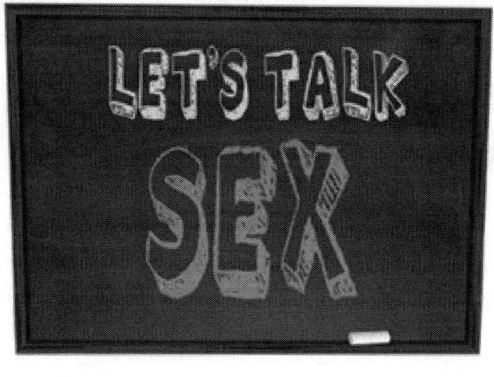

Slide 23

Sex Education

- Provided by someone with special expertise
- Children with disabilities have the right to the same education about sexuality as their peers
- May need modifications
  - Simplifying information
  - Using special teaching materials as needed
    - Anatomically correct dolls
    - Role-playing
    - Frequently reviewing and reinforcing the material
    - IEPs/IHPs should include provision of sexuality education

Black & Baker, 2013

Slide 24

Sex Education

- Remember this is developmental and questions are completely normal.
  - Sexual thoughts or actions are not negative risk behaviors.
- Parents/youth workers can help adolescents make safe and healthy choices regarding sexual behavior by:
  - Maintaining open lines of communication
  - Ensuring access to appropriate information and resources
  - Providing complete and accurate sex education so adolescents with IDD can make informed decisions
- A team process
  - Planned and coordinated by support team
  - Parent input
  - Not just DSP

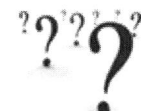

Black & Baker, 2013

Slide 25

Privacy

- Teach which behaviors are acceptable to do only when they are alone
  - Provide guidelines about when
  - Review expectations
  - Provide guidelines about where
  - Ensure the guidelines are followed
- Identify and recognize cues in the environment (a closed door)
- Social cues for public settings
- Create cues for alone time (a sign on the door)

Richards, et al, 2012

Slide 26

Working Together

- Empower young people to set limits.

- Assist lower-functioning individuals with achieving and maintaining privacy.

- When supervising or assisting with personal care:
  - Be considerate
  - Ask permission
  - Remember they still need privacy
  - Seek to minimize discomfort

Slide 27

Intimate Relationships

- Another important consideration is developing and maintaining intimate relationships.
  - Emotional intimacy
  - Physical intimacy

- Developmentally appropriate information about sexuality can help individuals with IDD attain a life with more personal fulfillment.

Walsh, Margaret

M
O
D
U
L
E

1
1

Slide 28

Sexual Orientation

- In addition to physical development of sexual characteristics, exploration of sexual orientation is a normal part of sexual development.

- Sexual orientation is the pattern of to whom one is physically and emotionally attracted. There is a growing list of terms used to describe one's sexual orientation, but the majority fall into one of the three following categories:
  - Heterosexuality (Straight)
  - Homosexuality (Gay/Lesbian)
  - Bisexuality

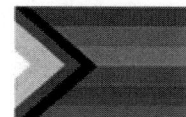

APA, 2008

Slide 29

Gender Identity

- Gender Identity – an individual's inherent sense of being male, female, a blend of male and female or an alternative gender.

- Transgender – when an individual's gender identity does not correspond with their biological sex.
  - Often beginning in youth
  - May or may not be presented outwardly for others to see

- Genderqueer/Gender-fluid/Non-Binary – those whose gender identity does not align with a binary understanding of gender

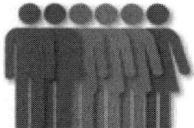

APA, 2015

Slide 30

Sexual Orientation and Gender Identity

- IDD + LGBTQ = greater risk of bullying and harassment

- Competent, compassionate care providers should be sought

- Access to the LGBTQ+ community

- Support from caregivers is vital

Walsh, Margaret

Slide 31

Peer Pressure

- Peer pressure is one thing all teens have in common.
  - Need for acceptance, approval and belonging is vital during the teen years.
  - Teens who feel isolated or rejected are more likely to engage in risky behaviors to fit in with a group.
- During adolescence, people begin to spend a lot more time with their friends and less time with their family.
  - More susceptible to the influences of their peers.

Slide 32

Peer Pressure

- Pressure isn't always negative.
  - Pressure into negative behaviors
  - Away from positive behaviors
  - Positive influences, such as doing well in school, having respect for others and avoiding taking negative risks
- Handling peer pressure depends largely on how adolescents feel about themselves.

Slide 33

Bullying

- Childhood bullies are more likely to become young adult criminals than are non-bullies. Bullied children may grow up with diminished self-confidence.
- Physical aggression: hitting, kicking, pushing, choking, punching.
- Verbal aggression: threatening, taunting, teasing, starting rumors, fostering fear, hate speech.
- Exclusion from activities.

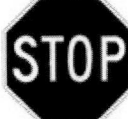

M O D U L E 1 1

Slide 34

Bullying

- Done by someone with more power or social support to someone with less power or social support.
- Often includes the abuser blaming the target for the abuse.
- Often leads to the target blaming him or herself for the abuse.
- In most bullying situations, the target cannot stop the bullying by his or her own actions.

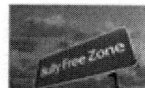

Slide 35

Exercise

- How do you think the way bullying is portrayed in popular TV shows/movies can affect a young person with IDD?

- What happened and how did the bullying resolve?

Slide 36

Stopping Bullying: What Doesn't Work

- **Denial:** ("She would never do that;" "I'm sure he didn't mean to hurt you;" "Boys are just like that;" "Sticks and stones may break bones, but words will never harm").
- **Telling the victim to solve the problem:** ("Just make sure you're never alone with that kid;" "Say no;" "Stand up for yourself and hit back;" "Wear less revealing clothes;" "Pretend it doesn't bother you").
- **Broad-brush educational efforts alone:** ("Soft is the heart of a child;" Sensitivity training; "Hands are for helping, not hurting").

Slide 37

Stopping Bullying: What Works

- Consistent enforcement of effective consequences that are predictable, inevitable, immediate and escalating.
- Monitoring to make sure consequences and education are effective.
- Effective counseling for youth who bully after enforcement of consequences has generated some anxiety.

Slide 38

Stopping Bullying: What Works

- Effective support for targets, including protection from repeat victimization.
- Empowering bystanders to tell adults, support targets and discourage unacceptable behavior.

Slide 39

Cyberbullying

Cyberbullying is bullying that takes place using electronic technology. Examples of cyberbullying include:

- Mean text messages or emails
- Rumors sent by email or posted on social networking sites
- Embarrassing pictures, videos, websites or fake profiles posted online

Baker, 2013

Slide 40

Why Cyberbullying is Different

- Cyberbullying can happen 24 hours a day, seven days a week, and reach a young person even when he or she is alone.
- Cyberbullying messages and images can be posted anonymously and distributed quickly to a very wide audience. It can be difficult and sometimes impossible to trace the source.
- Deleting inappropriate or harassing messages, texts and pictures is extremely difficult after they have been posted or sent.

Baker, 2013

Slide 41

How Much Does It Happen?

- The 2020 Indicators of School Crime and Safety (National Center for Education Statistics and Bureau of Justice Statistics) indicates that, nationwide, about 24 percent of students were in schools where bullying occurred at least monthly.
- The 2020 Indicators of School Crime and Safety (National Center for Education Statistics and Bureau of Justice Statistics) indicates that 15 percent of students experienced cyberbullying at least once a week. The cyberbullying summary shows 36.5 percent lifetime victimization rates.

Baker, 2013

Slide 42

How to Prevent Cyberbullying

- Be aware of online activity
- Monitor online activity
- Talk about online activity
- Teaching online safety
- Set rules

Baker, 2013

M
O
D
U
L
E

1
1

Slide 43

If Cyberbullying Occurs

- Keep evidence of the activity
- Don't respond
- Use blocking technology
- Report to service providers
- Report to law enforcement if appropriate
- Involve schools

Baker, 2013

Slide 44

Gangs

- Gang violence has spread to communities throughout the world. In the U.S., these are the statistics:
  - More than 24,500 different youth gangs around the country
  - More than 772,500 teens and young adult members
- Teens join gangs for a variety of reasons:
  - Seeking excitement
  - Looking for prestige
  - Protection
  - Make money
  - A sense of belonging
- Few teens are forced to join gangs; most can refuse to join without fear of retaliation.

Slide 45

Steps to Conflict Resolution

- **Set the stage.** Agree to try to work together to find a solution peacefully and establish ground rules (e.g., no name-calling, yelling, or interrupting).
- **Gather perspectives.** Each person describes his/her perspective. Listeners pay attention to what the others say they want and why.
- **Find common interests.** Establish points everyone agrees on. Identify common interests; can be as simple as a shared need to save face.
- **Create options.** Brainstorm possible solutions in which both people gain something. Think win-win!
- **Evaluate options.** Each teen discusses feelings about solutions. Negotiate to reach a conclusion acceptable to both.
- **Create an agreement.** The teens explicitly state their agreement and may even want to write it down.

Slide 46

Adolescent disorders

- Teens deal with related issues all the time; when it gets out of hand, then it's a disorder.
- May manifest differently than with adults.
- Common problems:
  - Eating disorders
  - Depression
  - Substance abuse

Slide 47

Eating Disorders

- Anorexia nervosa
  - Intense fear of becoming obese does not diminish as weight is lost.
  - Disturbed body image — claims to "feel fat" even when emaciated.
  - Loss of at least 25 percent of original body weight.
  - Refusal to maintain normal body weight.

- Bulimia
  - Recurrent episodes of binge-eating (rapidly consuming large amounts of food in a short time).
  - Often followed by purging via vomiting or laxatives.

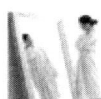

Slide 48

Eating Disorders: Causes and Solutions

- Causes
  - Adolescent focus on body image
  - Cultural emphasis on appearances
  - Other unmet emotional needs
- Response
  - Requires formal treatment
  - May include: lectures, group therapy, assertiveness training, drug therapy and nutritional counseling
- Cautions
  - Avoid arguing; you're not going to talk them out of it.
  - Be careful to avoid criticism.

Slide 49

Early Onset of Mental Illness

- Environmental stress does not cause mental illness but can trigger onset.
- Biological events, chemical imbalance or disturbance requires psychiatric treatment.
- Untreatable mental illness places children at the risk of developing severe forms as adults, more reluctant to seek proper treatment.
- Poor functioning in school, development, social relationships, family life.
- Therapy can support but is insufficient to treat many severe illness driven symptoms and behaviors.
- Observation is key to diagnosis: intensity, frequency, impact.

Slide 50

Triggers for Emotional Crises

- Onset of illness (medical or mental)
- Birth of sibling
- Onset of puberty/adolescence
- Start or end of school
- Out of home placement
- Sex and dating issues
- Changes in staff and teacher relationships

- Surpassed by younger siblings or peers
- Inappropriate expectations of others
- Physical, sexual or emotional abuse
- Illness/aging of parents
- Death of parent, caretaker or family member
- Loss of peer or roommate

Slide 51

Exercise

Consider wellness strategies you can use to support a young person with IDD who might experience one of the emotional crises listed on the previous slide. Discuss with the group.

MODULE 11

Slide 52

Child Adolescent Depression

- Not just bad moods and occasional sadness
- Serious problem that impacts every aspect of a teen's life
- Requires treatment and can lead to:
  - Problems at home and school
  - Drug abuse
  - Poor adjustment and self-image
  - Negative identity
  - Homicide, violence or suicide

Slide 53

Depression Signs and Symptoms

- Sadness or hopelessness
- Irritability, anger or hostility
- Tearfulness or frequent crying
- Withdrawal from friends and family
- Loss of interest in activities
- Changes in eating and sleeping habits
- Restlessness and agitation
- Feelings of worthlessness and guilt

Slide 54

Depression Signs and Symptoms

- Lack of enthusiasm and motivation
- Fatigue or lack of energy
- Difficulty concentrating
- Thoughts of death or suicide
- Physical complaints (far more likely in youth than adults)

Slide 55

Warning Signs of Teen Suicide

- Talking or joking about suicide.
- Saying things like "I'd be better off dead" or "I wish I could disappear forever."
- Speaking positively about death or romanticizing dying ("If I died, people might love me more").
- Writing stories and poems about death or dying.

Slide 56

Warning Signs of Teen Suicide

- Engaging in reckless behavior or having a lot of accidents resulting in injury.
- Giving away prized possessions.
- Saying goodbye to friends and family in dramatic ways.
- Seeking out weapons, pills or other ways to kill themselves.

Slide 57

Talking Tips for Depressed Teens

- Offer support
  - Let them know you're there for them. Avoid asking lots of questions (teens don't like to feel patronized).
  - Make it clear you're ready and willing to provide whatever support they need.
- Be gentle but persistent
  - Don't give up if they shut you out.
  - Talking about depression can be very tough for teens.
  - Be respectful; show you are concerned and willing to listen.

Slide 58

Talking Tips for Depressed Teens

- Listen without lecturing
  - Resist criticizing or passing judgment; when they talk, at least they are communicating.
  - Avoid offering unsolicited advice.
- Validate feelings
  - Don't try to talk them out of depression.
  - Acknowledge the pain and sadness they are feeling.
  - Make them feel like you take their emotions seriously.

Slide 59

Substance Abuse

- Experimenting
  - Teens may try alcohol, cigarettes, inhalants or other drugs one or more times but not go any further.
  - Usually do not have any problems as a result of substance use.
- Substance abuse
  - Experimenting leads to regular or frequent use.
  - Substance abuse results in problems at home (more arguments), at school (such as failing grades) or with the law.
- Substance dependence (addiction)
  - Physical and/or psychological dependence.
  - Use takes up a significant portion of the teen's activities.
  - Continues despite causing harm and is difficult to stop.
  - An ongoing, and possibly fatal, disease.

Slide 60

Health Care

- Adolescents — facilitate a transition to more active role in healthy behavior, medication management, appointments.
- Help young people to understand their disability or diagnosis and health concerns.
- Identify reliable resources for further information
- Teach healthy lifestyle skills, promote wellness.
- Empower them to be more involved in asking questions and making decisions.
- Provide guidance in knowing how and when to acquire or decline further help and support.

Slide 61

Community Safety

- Who/what is dangerous?
  - Help identify potential danger and make decisions beforehand about safety and trust.
  - Build awareness by reviewing everyday dangers often: fire safety, traffic, crime, internet threats, risk-taking behavior.
  - Build confidence to act safely "in the moment."
    - Discuss potentially threatening situations.
    - Practice or role-play appropriate response.
    - Review who/how to ask for help.

Slide 62

Safety Tips

- Teach the person to always let someone know where he/she is going and for how long.
- Routines
  - Many children with IDD depend on routines.
  - Avoid routines that others can predict to victimize children.
- Talk about safety often.

Slide 63

Potential Victimization

- Appearance of safety doesn't mean there is no threat.

- Grooming — The establishment of trust through repeated interaction to increase access to a potential victim and decrease likelihood of discovery.

- Awareness
  - Can children recognize they are being "set up"?
  - Are parents/care providers able to tell when children don't see it?
  - What "Don't talk to strangers" means.

Slide 64

Internet Safety

- Keep the computer in a high-traffic area.
- Monitor use of other digital devices.
- Establish limits for which online sites children may visit and for how long.
- Remember that Internet technology can be mobile, so make sure to monitor cell phones, gaming devices and laptops.
- Surf the Internet with children and let them show you what they like to do online.
- Ask questions about their interests and have them show you what they are searching.
- Bookmark/shortcuts to apps and safe websites for immediate access.
- Continually dialogue with children about online safety.

Slide 65

Technology Safety

- Know who young people are communicating with online.
- Note numbers of outgoing/incoming calls with no contact information.
- Open a family/group/house email account to share with younger children.
- Brainstorm screen names and email addresses that do not contain information about gender, identity or location and avoid being suggestive.

Slide 66

More Technology Safety

- Teach children never to open emails/messages from unknown senders and to use settings to block messages from people they do not know.
- Be aware of other ways children may be going online — with cell phones, laptops, tablets, games or from friends' homes or the library.
- Remind children that anything they send from their phones can be easily forwarded and shared.
- Familiarize yourself with popular acronyms at sites like netlingo.com and noslang.com.

Slide 67

Social Networking: Benefits

Gain social confidence and become more secure in new situations, such as going to college, joining a sports team and meeting new friends.

Learn about his or her diagnosis and health needs.

Find support in online communities — especially true for kids who have unique interests or feel isolated.

Make friends who are interested in the same things or may be dealing with similar issues.

Slide 68

Social Networking: More Benefits

Keep in touch with family members who live far away by sharing updates, photos, videos and messages.

Be creative sharing ideas or through poetry, blogging or journaling.

Increasing media literacy and expand vocabulary and communication skills.

Generate topics for discussion in "live" conversations and with peers in school and other offline settings.

Slide 69

Supporting Young People to Develop Goals

Set realistic expectations by considering:
- Strengths, abilities and interests.
- Opportunities, resources and feasibility.

Be careful not to devalue someone's ambitions.

Break larger goals into mini-goals or objectives.
- See progress quickly.
- Even on a daily basis if needed.

Establish incentives that are meaningful to the person.

Be flexible. Use setbacks as building blocks to modify goals or create new dreams (turn disappointment into opportunity).

Post-test

Module XI: Childhood and Adolescence

_____ 1. Functioning and behavior are influenced by:
(a) The Eltdown gland
(b) Stages of development
(c) A static pathway all young people follow
(d) None of the above

_____ 2. Cultural perspectives of the family must:
(a) Always be taken into account
(b) Sometimes be taken into account
(c) Never be taken into account
(d) Be considered only when they clash with treatment goals

_____ 3. One of the first people to study the development of a personal identity was:
(a) Randolph Carter
(b) Tara Maclay
(c) B.F. Skinner
(d) Erik Erikson

_____ 4. A sense of identity includes:
(a) Gender identity
(b) Sense of purpose
(c) Knowledge of character traits
(d) All of the above

_____ 5. Which of the following is not true about most cases of bullying?
(a) It's done by someone with more power or social support to someone with less power or social support
(b) It often includes the abuser blaming the target for the abuse
(c) It often leads to vengeance spells
(d) In most bullying situations, the target cannot stop the bullying by their own actions

_____ 6. Cyberbullying is:
(a) Becoming less common quickly due to efforts by social media companies
(b) Difficult to prosecute due to the court case Gibbous vs. Pnakotic
(c) Likely to cause real-world problems for targets
(d) Not a big worry because it is all online anyway

_____ 7. Which of the following is not a common adolescent problem?
(a) Senescence
(b) Eating disorders
(c) Depression
(d) Substance abuse

_____ 8. Which of the following is an eating disorder?
(a) Anorexia nervosa
(b) Bulimia
(c) Both (a) and (b)
(d) Neither (a) or (b)

_____ 9. Substance dependence is an extra concern for youth with IDD due to:
(a) Lack of understanding of long-term consequences
(b) Greater access to street drugs than typical youth
(c) Higher risk of physical dependence than typical youth
(d) All of the above

_____ 10. What is the best way to help a young person with IDD be safe in the community?
(a) Use Hazred's decision matrix
(b) Teach the young person who and what can be dangerous
(c) Follow the same routines always, as that builds comfort
(d) Look for the appearance of safety

MODULE 11

Supplemental Materials

Module XI: Childhood and Adolescence

Come up with 10 words that describe you.

1. _____

2. _____

3. _____

4. _____

5. _____

6. _____

7. _____

8. _____

9. _____

10. _____

Now, **circle** the ones that are related to work. Put a **star** next to the ones that will never, ever change no matter what.

Risk-Taking

This module presents risk-taking as a normal part of life and development. Make your own list of unhealthy and healthy risks, in addition to the ones on the slides.

Unhealthy risks	Healthy risks

What are healthy risks you personally take?

_____

_____

What are some healthy risks you see among people you support?

_____

_____

Sexuality and Gender

What have you learned about sexual and gender expression among people you support?

_____

_____

How does a person with intellectual or developmental disabilities differ from typical people in sexual and gender expression?

M
O
D
U
L
E

1
1

_____

_____

Bullying

Bullying is a significant concern in childhood and adolescence. We discuss it in great detail in this module. Have you seen bullying outside of your work?

_____

_____

Have you seen people with intellectual or developmental disabilities be bullied?

_____

_____

What is your experience with cyberbullying?

_____

_____

Are people you support online or on virtual platforms where cyberbullying might occur?

_____

_____

Emotional Crises

What are the triggers for emotional crises that you have seen among people you support?

_____

_____

M
O
D
U
L
E

1
1

What do emotional crises look like? Describe some you have seen.

_____

_____

What wellness strategies could you use to support a young person with IDD who might experience an emotional crisis?

_____

_____

If a person you support tells you they are feeling really blue, what might you say back?

_____

_____

Internet and Technology

This module shares ideas for safe use of technology. Which of the tips on Internet safety might you use in supporting people?

_____

_____

Do you practice technology safety?

_____

_____

M O D U L E 1 1

Social Networking

What are the good things about social networking?	What are the bad things about social networking?

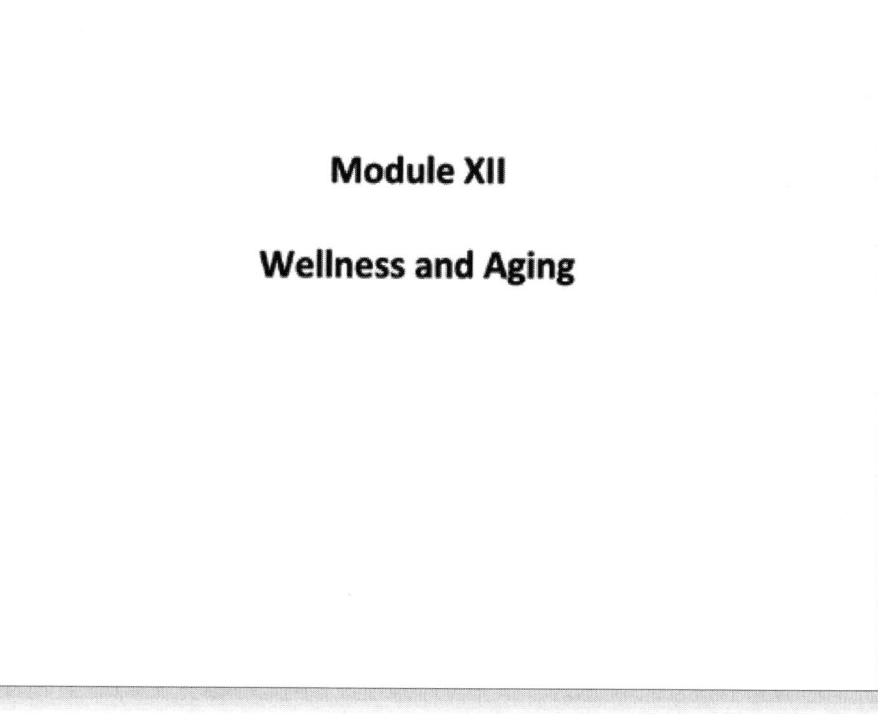

Module XII

Wellness and Aging

Pre-test

Module XII: Wellness and Aging

_____ 1.   True or false: Older people with IDD generally have poorer health, greater need for support and experience greater health-related functional decline than do older people without IDD.

_____ 2.   Life expectancy for people with Down syndrome has _____ in recent decades.
(a) Remained the same
(b) Increased dramatically
(c) Decreased dramatically
(d) Decreased slightly

_____ 3.   True or false: Older adults are not able to learn new material or remember new things as they age.

_____ 4.   Some factors that might affect aging in people with IDD include:
(a) Genetics
(b) Lifestyle
(c) Health
(d) All of the above

_____ 5.   _____ is a technique or modification to our behavior or environment that we use to compensate for a deficit, weakness, injury or perceived inadequacy in a specific area or skill.
(a) Sensory changes
(b) Compensatory strategy
(c) Dementia
(d) Memory

_____ 6.   Which of the following sensory changes can be associated with aging?
(a) Decreased social isolation
(b) Increased attention span
(c) Increase in falls
(d) None of the above

_____ 7. Some helpful interventions to create a supportive environment and increase comfort include:
(a) Minimize the time aging people spend in the community
(b) Provide proper lighting, reduce background noise and minimize clutter, such as rugs
(c) Introduce new food and people to the environment
(d) Encourage older people to retire

_____ 8. Which of the following is not a negative social aspect of aging?
(a) Cognitive decline
(b) Grief and loss
(c) Travel
(d) Accepting mortality

_____ 9. _____ is a legal document in which a person specifies what actions should be taken for their health if they are no longer able to make decisions for themselves because of illness or incapacity.
(a) An advance healthcare directive
(b) Wellness plan
(c) Primary care toolkit
(d) A compensatory strategy

_____ 10. Wellness recommendations identified as those with the greatest potential for changing or improving healthy aging include:
(a) Promoting health and preventing illness/injury
(b) Optimizing mental and physical health
(c) Managing chronic conditions
(d) All of the above

MODULE 12

Slide 1

Module XII

Wellness and Aging

Slide 2

The purpose of this module is to discuss mental wellness among persons with IDD who are aging, considering the experiences of typical persons as well and how best to address their changing support needs.

Slide 3

Learning Objectives

- Describe the age-related health problems attributed to people with IDD, including dementia and the challenges in diagnosing.
- Describe the psycho-social aspects of aging with IDD and how to support a person to maintain healthy psycho-social contacts.
- Identify how to enhance supports in consideration of health and wellness factors affecting people with IDD as they age.

MODULE 12

Slide 4

The WHO (World Health Organization) acknowledges that aging is a lifelong process of change and there is no generally accepted age that defines exactly when people become old.

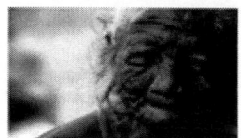

WHO, 2000

Slide 5

Understanding Aging

For some people, the types of changes that occur toward the end of their lives may require more care and support.

As people who have a dual diagnosis age, understanding and supporting their mental wellness is crucial.

Slide 6

A New Perspective

Clinical definition: "Aging is a continuation of the developmental process and is influenced by genetic and other biological factors as well as personal and social circumstances."

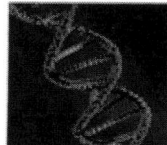

Holland, 2000

Slide 7

A Diverse Process

The accumulation of changes over time occur at different rates depending on an individual's genetics, environment and lifestyle.

Physical and physiological changes make the body more susceptible to illness, but no certain pathology is predictable without consideration of lifestyle variables (Saxon et al., 2009).

Slide 8

Exercise

What words come to your mind when you hear the word "aging"?

Slide 9

Aging and IDD

Due to factors associated with their disabilities and other health disparities, people with IDD generally have poorer health, greater need for support and experience greater health-related functional decline than do older people without IDD.

Bigby, 2004

Slide 10

For some people who have IDD, aging can be complicated by the occurrence of what appears to be premature aging and shortened life expectancy, particularly for people with profound and multiple disabilities and frequently those with Down syndrome.

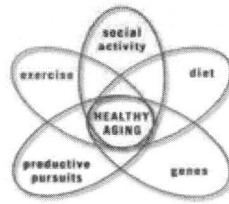

Slide 11

Aging in the General Population

Aging in the general population increases vulnerability to certain health issues:

- Memory and Alzheimer's disease
- Sensory problems: eye and ear conditions
- Digestive and metabolic disorders
- Urogenital conditions such as incontinence and prostate cancer
- Dental conditions such as periodontitis, gingivitis and tooth loss
- Skin conditions such as skin cancers, shingles, dry skin, pruritus, geriatric eczema

NIH, 2007

Slide 12

Concepts in Physical Aging

Skeletal system

Nervous system

Physical abilities are compromised

NIH, 2007

Slide 13

Learning and Memory

Common myths and stereotypes have long implied that older adults are not able to learn new material or that poor memory is part of aging (Saxon et al., 2009).

People continue to have different
learning styles as they age.

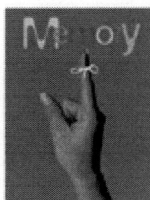

Slide 14

Life Expectancy

As a result of advances in health care and community supports, life expectancy is increasing for people who have intellectual/developmental disabilities.

For example, life expectancy for people with Down syndrome has increased dramatically in recent decades, from 25 in 1983 to 60 today.

Bigby, 2004

Slide 15

The Differences in Aging with an IDD

- Genetics
- Environmental factors and lifestyle
- Access to specialized health and mental health services for people who have IDD or dual diagnosis
- Communication
- Accelerated aging

Baxter et al, 2006 and Ringaert and Waters, 2005

Slide 16

Accelerated Physical Aging

There is evidence that people with IDD develop secondary conditions and diseases. As a result, they may age at a different rate than the general population.

Features of aging that can manifest as a gradual reduction in ability or capacity in an individual in the general population can occur more rapidly in someone with IDD.

Kailes, 2006

Slide 17

Other age-related health issues are more frequent in people with particular genetically based syndromes.

- Mitral valve prolapse and musculoskeletal disorders in people with Fragile X syndrome.
- Scoliosis in people with Prader-Willi syndrome.
- Recurrent upper respiratory and ear infections in people with Cri-du-Chat syndrome.

Temkin, 2009

Slide 18

For many intellectual/developmental disabilities with genetic etiology, there are known, existing predispositions for specified medical, mental health and behavioral challenges.

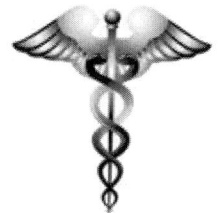

Sullivan et al, 2011

M
O
D
U
L
E

1
2

Slide 19

The most commonly known of these is the increased risk of precocious aging, dementia and increased sensory loss in people with Down syndrome.

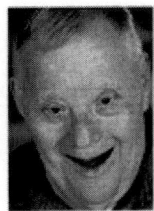

Wishart, 1998

Slide 20

Sensory Changes and Aging

- Reduced acuity and alertness
- Increased masking and compensatory strategies
- Reduced potential for independence
- Increased social isolation
- Decreased attention span
- Increase in falls

Slide 21

Exercise

A **compensatory strategy** is a technique or modification to our behavior or environment that we use to compensate for a deficit, weakness, injury or perceived inadequacy in a specific area or skill.

Activity: Think of a compensatory strategy you use when you run into someone whose name you forgot or when you set a new security password to remember.

Discussion: In the same circumstances, would that compensatory strategy potentially be different for a person who has an IDD?

Slide 22

The prevalence of certain mental health issues increases with aging, including anxiety, depression, dementia and psychosis.

From the available research, it can be reasonably concluded that people who have IDD are more likely to develop a mental health issue as they age.

Patel, Goldberg & Moss, 1993

Slide 23

Prevalence of Mental Health Problems

The rate of psychiatric problems for people who have IDD is two to four times the rate of the general population as they age.

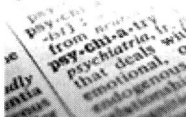

Torr & Davis, 2007

Slide 24

Dementia

The DSM-5 defines dementia as Neurocognitive Disorder. It involves the "loss of memory plus impairment in at least one other cognitive function, such as aphasia, apraxia, agnosia; and disturbance in executive function, which is severe enough to interfere with activities of daily living and represents a decline."

APA, 2000, 2013

Slide 25

Dementia Prevalence Rate

- 22 percent of adults 40+ who have Down syndrome develop dementia.

- The rate increases to 56 percent for adults 60+.

- For individuals with other types of IDD, the rate is comparable to that of the general population: 5 percent in adults 60+.

Janicki & Dalton, 2000 and Fletcher, et al., 2007

Slide 26

Challenges in Diagnosing Dementia

- Measuring decline in functioning
- Self-reporting observations
- No standardized criteria for dementia

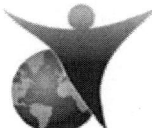

Cooper, 1997

Slide 27

Diagnostic Overshadowing & Misdiagnosis

- Assumption that lack of cognition or sensory changes are due to IDD or MI
- Age-associated changes that may be misidentified as dementia:
    - Adjustment: grief and loss
    - Dehydration, constipation, nutritional imbalances
    - Sleep challenges
    - Visual impairments, cataracts, glaucoma
    - Urinary discomfort, UTIs

Slide 28

Case illustration: Maria is a woman with Down syndrome. She is in her 40s and her health is failing. She suffers from digestive discomfort and sometimes has trouble hearing. She no longer has the energy to do the things she likes to do, and her favorite TV show, *The Office,* has gone off the air. Her life just seems to be slipping away. She gets crabby and takes her frustration out on staff, taking an occasional swing when she has energy and spitting at staff when she does not.

Exercise: Think about ways you could use these approaches to develop interventions to support Maria's wellness: positive behavior supports, mental health interventions and person-centered planning.

Slide 29

For people who have an intellectual/developmental disability, lifelong attention to preventable medical and mental health conditions is critical for healthy aging.

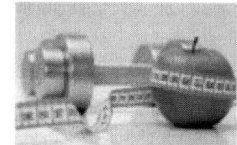

Slide 30

Best Practice Guidelines for Physicians

In 2011, Canadian Consensus Guidelines were developed for primary care physicians on evidence-based best practice in preventative health care for people with IDD.

In 2014, these tools were adapted by Vanderbilt Kennedy University Center for Excellence in Developmental Disabilities for use within the U.S. health care system.

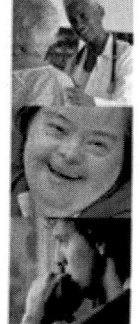

Slide 31

Primary Care Toolkit

The Canadian Primary Care Guidelines and Toolkit are available at: https://www.cna-aiic.ca/en/nursing-practice/tools-for-practice/primary-care-toolkit

The primary care tools adapted for use in the US health care system are available at: https://iddtoolkit.vkcsites.org/

Slide 32

Creating a Supportive Setting

Confusing surroundings can be unsafe and frustrating for people as they age. Creating a supportive environment and addressing potential issues can help minimize changes and provide comfort.

Slide 33

Creating a Supportive Setting

- Proper lighting
- Bold colors
- Reduce background noise
- Increase visual aids
- Non-slip surfaces
- Remove rugs
- Reduce clutter

- Check water and climate temperature
- Gentle soaps
- More seasoned food
- Visual aids
- Smoke detectors
- Clearly marked exits
- Rounded furniture

Adapted from Gilbride, M 2016

Slide 34

Activity: Help Tom

Tom has Down syndrome and has been experiencing early signs of dementia. He's been having trouble at mealtimes: He can eat finger foods, but he can't find food on the plate with his fork. And when he gets up to use the bathroom at night, he cannot find his way back to his room.

Help Tom using some ideas on the previous slide or your own.

Slide 35

The Social Aspects of Aging

As with all people, aging people with IDD deal with a variety of psycho-social changes and support as they age.

*   Increasing social isolation
*   Changing interests
*   Declining energy
*   Retirement

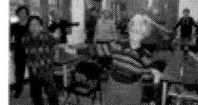

Temkin, 2009

Slide 36

The Social Aspects of Aging

*   Cognitive decline
*   Financial and estate management
*   Loss of family and friends
*   Grief management
*   Acceptance of mortality
*   Lack of meaningful work or hobbies

Temkin, 2009

Slide 37

Social Value

Social value contributes to overall wellness for all people.

This includes people who have IDD who want to participate in and contribute to their communities in the same manner as all citizens.

Slide 38

Exercise

What social value did you experience from older people as you were growing up?

- Did you spend time around your grandparents?
- Were older people respected during your childhood?
- How can we ensure the people with IDD can continue to offer social value as they age?

Slide 39

Wellness

Wellness encompasses many components including:

- Promoting health and preventing illness, disease and injury.
- Optimizing mental and physical health.
- Managing chronic conditions.
- Engaging with life.

WHO, 2000

MODULE 12

Slide 40

Wellness

Key responsibilities for primary care and specialist health services:

1. Maintenance of the physical and mental health of people with IDD

2. Early detection and treatment of both physical and mental health problems

Poindexter, 2002

Slide 41

Working Together

As people who have IDD age, there is ongoing need for collaborative supports and services to address the needs of the person in this stage of life to ensure that wellness is assured as an accepted part of aging for this population.

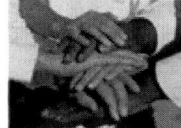

Slide 42

End-of-Life Considerations

- Thinking ahead matters.
- Identify a person who will act in the best interest of the individual. Consider someone in his/her social or spiritual community.
- Help people understand there are options to plan for treatment, at a time when they might be unable to make informed decisions (advance directives, health care proxy, substitute decision-maker or power of attorney).

MODULE 12

Slide 43

Advance Care Planning

Advance care planning involves learning about the types of decisions that might need to be made, considering those decisions ahead of time and then letting others know your preferences.

It is important to engage people with IDD in supported decision-making about end-of-life issues.

Learn more at:
nia.nih.gov/health/advance-care-planning-healthcare-directives

Slide 44

Advance Care Directive

- An advance healthcare directive, also known as a medical directive, is a legal document in which a person specifies what actions should be taken for their health if they are no longer able to make decisions for themselves because of illness or incapacity.
- In the United States, each state regulates the use of advance directives differently. A living will is one type of advance directive. It takes effect when the patient is terminally ill.

Slide 45

Power of Attorney

A "durable power of attorney for health care" is also called a "health care power of attorney." It's a legal document in which a person names a proxy (agent) to make all health care decisions if one becomes unable to do so.

A proxy or, substitute decision-maker, also known as a representative, surrogate or agent, should be familiar with the person's values and wishes. This means he or she will be able to decide when treatment decisions need to be made. A proxy can be chosen in addition to or instead of a living will.

Slide 46

- In Canada, a similar document is called a "power of attorney for personal care or for property." To be able to appoint a power of attorney, the person must be considered capable of making their own decisions around care and finances. This can be a challenge for people who have moderate to severe IDD. In these situations, decisions around care and finance may be made by an appropriate, identified substitute decision-maker. Separate acts govern substitute decision-making in each province and territory. For more information, search substitute decision-making for your province or territory.

- The Advance Care Planning in Canada: A National Framework and Implementation Project

Slide 47

Resources & Publications

Complex moral issues: End-of-life decisions for adults with significant intellectual disabilities.
ucedd.georgetown.edu/complex/

A caregiver's guide to the dying process.
hospicefoundation.org/HFA-Products/Caregiver-s-Guide-to-the-Dying-Process

The Center for Excellence in Aging & Community Wellness (CEACW)
A guide for supporting older people with intellectual disabilities and their families.
ceacw.org/

Slide 48

Resources & Publications

Options and Decision-Making at End of Life—Canada
canada.ca/en/health-canada/services/options-decision-making-end-life.html

Advance Care Planning—Canada
https://www.advancecareplanning.ca/resources-and-tools/

Powers of Attorney—Canada
canada.ca/en/employment-social-development/corporate/seniors/forum/power-attorney-financial.html

MODULE 12

Post-test

Module XII: Wellness and Aging

_____ 1.   True or false: Older people with IDD generally have poorer health, greater need for support and experience greater health-related functional decline than do older people without IDD.

_____ 2.   Life expectancy for people with Down syndrome has _____ in recent decades.
(a) Remained the same
(b) Increased dramatically
(c) Decreased dramatically
(d) Decreased slightly

_____ 3.   True or false: Older adults are not able to learn new material or remember new things as they age.

_____ 4.   Some factors that might affect aging in people with IDD include:
(a) Genetics
(b) Lifestyle
(c) Health
(d) All of the above

_____ 5.   _____ is a technique or modification to our behavior or environment that we use to compensate for a deficit, weakness, injury or perceived inadequacy in a specific area or skill.
(a) Sensory changes
(b) Compensatory strategy
(c) Dementia
(d) Memory

_____ 6.   Which of the following sensory changes can be associated with aging?
(a) Decreased social isolation
(b) Increased attention span
(c) Increase in falls
(d) None of the above

_____ 7. Some helpful interventions to create a supportive environment and increase comfort include:

(a) Minimize the time aging people spend in the community

(b) Provide proper lighting, reduce background noise and minimize clutter, such as rugs

(c) Introduce new food and people to the environment

(d) Encourage older people to retire

_____ 8. Which of the following is not a negative social aspect of aging?

(a) Cognitive decline

(b) Grief and loss

(c) Travel

(d) Accepting mortality

_____ 9. _____ is a legal document in which a person specifies what actions should be taken for their health if they are no longer able to make decisions for themselves because of illness or incapacity.

(a) An advance healthcare directive

(b) Wellness plan

(c) Primary care toolkit

(d) A compensatory strategy

_____ 10. Wellness recommendations identified as those with the greatest potential for changing or improving healthy aging include:

(a) Promoting health and preventing illness/injury

(b) Optimizing mental and physical health

(c) Managing chronic conditions

(d) All of the above

MODULE 12

Supplemental Materials

Module XII: Wellness and Aging

When you hear the word *aging*, what are some other words that come to mind? Try to list 10.

1. _____

2. _____

3. _____

4. _____

5. _____

6. _____

7. _____

8. _____

9. _____

10. _____

Below are some sensory changes people may experience as they age. Consider someone you support with IDD. Provide an example of behavior change you've noticed related to aging in the following areas.

Sensory Changes	Observation/Behavior
Reduced acuity (perception) and alertness	
Increased masking and compensatory strategies	
Reduced potential for independence	
Increased social isolation	
Decreased attention span	
Increase in falls	

A **compensatory strategy** is a technique to help perform tasks or skills that may be diminished by a limitation in a specific area. These methods can help people who have memory challenges due to aging, Alzheimer's, dementia, brain injury or other reasons.

Let's practice: What are some compensatory strategies that may help?

1. Irene is having difficulty remembering the days and times of her appointments.

    _____

    _____

2. Franco gets disoriented in the grocery store when he can't find an item he needs.

    _____

    _____

3. Helena forgets to renew her medications, so she is often left without her pills.

    _____

    _____

MODULE 12

Tips to Create a Supportive Setting to Address Aging Issues

Consider how you can implement these things for people you support to create comfortable, safe, predictable environments. Make a plan to do this with your team.

- Proper lighting

- Bold colors

- Reduce background noise

- Increase visual aids

- Non-slip surfaces

- Remove rugs

- Reduce clutter

- Check water and climate temperature

- Gentle soaps

- (Naturally) seasoned food

- Visual aids

- Smoke detectors

- Clearly marked exits

- Rounded furniture (no sharp edges)

Below are some social aspects of aging people may experience. Consider someone you support with IDD who may be experiencing behavioral and mental health changes. Provide an example of a wellness support you can provide that can lead to improved outcomes.

Social Aspects	Observation/Behavior
Cognitive decline	
Financial and estate management	
Loss of family and friends	
Grief management	
Acceptance of mortality	
Lack of meaningful work or hobbies	

Reflection

What social value did you experience from older people as you were growing up? Did you spend time around your grandparents or other older relatives during your childhood?

How can you ensure the people you support with IDD continue to offer social value as they age? Think about the things they value and what people value about them. Write some ideas below.

M
O
D
U
L
E

1
2

Resources

Older adults should consider planning ahead for end-of-life care and health crises. Here are resources and tools to help aging adults consider, prepare and communicate these decisions.

- Aging and Disability: Celebration of Life Checklist:
  http://www.aging-and-disability.org/documents/celebration_of_life_checklist.pdf

- Aging and Disability: Making an End of Life Plan:
  http://www.aging-and-disability.org/documents/making_an_end_of_life_plan.pdf

- My Life, My Wishes, Sharing My Journey:
  https://sonoranucedd.fcm.arizona.edu/publications/1275

Supporting people through grief and loss is an essential support of aging. Below are some further resources and tools.

- IDD/MH Grief & Loss Prescriber Guidelines:
  https://centerforstartservices.org/IDD-MH-Prescribing-Guidelines/grief

- Ritualizing Grief with People with IDD:
  https://rwjms.rutgers.edu/boggscenter/links/documents/RitualizingGriefIDD.pdf

- Helping People with IDD Process Grief:
  https://rwjms.rutgers.edu/boggscenter/links/documents/HelpingGriefIDD.pdf

- "My Goodbye Book" journal by Dr. Karyn Harvey:
  https://thenadd.org/wp-content/uploads/2019/10/my-goodbye-book.pdf

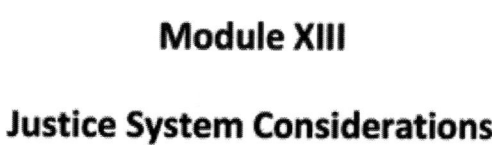

Module XIII

Justice System Considerations

Pre-test

Module XIII: Justice System Considerations

_____ 1. True or false: In the early part of the twentieth century, it was an accepted theory that people who have an intellectual/developmental disability were inherently criminal in their nature.

_____ 2. This is not a reason there are challenges in capturing accurate prevalence rates of people who have an intellectual/developmental disability who interact with the justice system:
(a) Underreporting to police services
(b) Stats tend to represent the arrest and conviction rate as opposed to the true offending prevalence
(c) People with IDD rarely get arrested
(d) Research more often focuses on the rates of recidivism as opposed to the rates of offending

_____ 3. Counterfeit criminality is:
(a) The concept that criminal behavior is performed for reasons other than criminality or criminal gain
(b) The concept that a person with IDD can appear innocent even if they are guilty of committing a crime
(c) When someone is falsely accused of a crime
(d) The same as bait-and-switch, which is unethical but not always illegal

_____ 4. Which of the following is not considered an effective means to support people who have IDD in avoiding criminal behavior?
(a) Assist people in developing friendships and learning about different types of social interactions
(b) Ensure people are aware of the laws in their state/province so they can avoid breaking the law
(c) Ensure people have an opportunity to advocate for themselves in ways they want
(d) Provide an opportunity for people to practice social skills in a variety of situations and environments

_____ 5. True or false: A person who has IDD frequently has specific vulnerabilities that can lead to initial involvement with the justice system and faces challenges that can often make it difficult to end that involvement or avoid future involvement.

_____ 6. When people who have an IDD become involved with the justice system, they frequently experience prejudice, lack of understanding and fear. They often experience difficulties with:
(a) Not being recognized as having a disability
(b) Being victimized at high rates
(c) Being denied opportunities for reparation
(d) All of the above
(e) (a) and (c) only

_____ 7. Fill in the blank: Fitness to stand trial, or _____ , refers to the ability of a person accused to participate in their own defense.

_____ 8. Forensic psychiatry relates to:
(a) Understanding the behavior and motivation of people who commit homicide
(b) Assessment and treatment of dangerous psychopaths
(c) The assessment, treatment and rehabilitation of people with serious mental illness who have come in contact with the law as a result of committing a crime
(d) The gathering and analysis of all crime-related psychological and psychiatric evidence in order to come to a conclusion about a suspect

_____ 9. True or false: A diagnosis of IDD and a mental illness means a person will be found unfit to stand trial.

_____ 10. Which of the following is not an ethical consideration that should be discussed before caregivers and service providers develop crisis plans that include calling police services:
(a) Is it the responsibility of the provider to manage aggressive behavior?
(b) Should a person who has IDD be charged for aggression to caregivers or providers?
(c) What is the goal of the intervention?
(d) What is the caregiver's or service provider's expectation of police services?
(e) None of the above

M
O
D
U
L
E

1
3

Slide 1

Module XIII

Justice System Considerations

Slide 2

This module contains information about the justice system as it relates to involvement with people who have an intellectual/developmental disability.

The goal is to assist service providers and clinicians to become more familiar with the system as they advocate for people with IDD who may become involved with justice.

Slide 3

Learning Objectives

- Understand the historical perspective on IDD and criminal behavior.
- Be aware of the vulnerabilities that can lead to involvement with the justice system.
- Recognize support needs of persons with IDD involved with the justice system.

Slide 4

Through the early part of the twentieth century, it was accepted theory that people with intellectual/developmental disabilities were inherently criminal in their behavior and their nature.

In fact, there is evidence that the belief in the criminal nature of people with IDD was a primary contributor to the move to institutional living and mass sterilization.

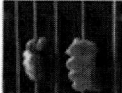

Luckasson (1988)

Slide 5

The middle to latter part of the twentieth century brought different theories about IDD and behavior in general, leading to a more balanced understanding today.

There is no greater propensity to criminal behavior for a person with IDD than for a person without IDD.

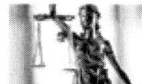

Bright (1989)

Slide 6

Prevalence Rates

Studies report a large range of estimates, from 2 percent to 40 percent, depending on methodology and diagnostic approach.

There is no strong evidence for different patterns of offending across types of abilities and disabilities.

Lindsay, Law & MacLeod (2002)

MODULE 13

Slide 7

Prevalence Rates

Establishing accurate or exact prevalence rates for specific conditions can be more effectively done depending on the visibility of the condition and the specific training provided to justice professionals around identification.

Lindsay, Law & MacLeod (2002)

Slide 8

Prevalence rates of people with IDD involved with the criminal justice system as the accused typically range between 1 to 8 percent.

- Data from police screening for mental disorders reported that 8 percent answered one of the four questions affirmatively; 96% percent reported reading and writing difficulty.

Goldman and Griffiths (2017)

Slide 9

Of those screened by police services:
  - 45 percent considered themselves to have a disability.
  - 40 percent had attended a special school.
  - 13 percent reported a coexisting mental health problem.
- Up to 24 percent of defendants in the criminal justice system may have intellectual disability.
- Rates in the prison population ranged from 0 to 9.5 percent.

Goldman and Griffiths (2017)

Slide 10

Counterfeit criminality refers to the concept in which criminal behavior is performed for reasons other than criminality or criminal gain.

Reasons include group membership or acceptance, the need to please peers, misunderstanding of the motives of others and the inability to see a setup.

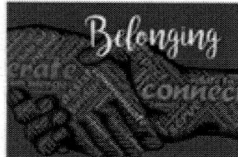

Hingsburger (2011)

Slide 11

Vulnerabilities

- More susceptible to being "the fall guy" or doing something illegal to impress someone else or make friends.
- When questioned by police, may not understand questions asked or their rights.
- More likely to confess to crimes they did not commit.
- Past experience may lead them to believe that if they agree, people will usually leave them alone.

Luckasson (1992)

Slide 12

Vulnerabilities

- People with IDD are more often held in custody pre-trial due to the inability to follow recognizance orders.
- People with IDD are often on a fixed income and have few family ties or limited social support, which means they have difficulty securing funds for surety or bail.
- If a person is supported by a community-based organization, the organization cannot act as surety or secure bail on the person's behalf.

Luckasson (1992)

Slide 13

Vulnerabilities

- People with IDD are more likely to be disciplined when in custody due to an inability to understand or follow institutional rules.
- People with IDD are more likely to have difficulty with others in custody due to an inability to understand institutional hierarchy or social rules.
- Frustration, fear or anxiety may manifest as challenging behavior that can lead to additional charges, the use of segregation and longer sentences.

Luckasson (1992)

Slide 14

When people who have IDD become involved with the justice system, they frequently experience prejudice, lack of understanding and fear. They often experience difficulties with:

- Not being recognized as having a disability
- Being victimized at high rates
- Being denied opportunities for reparation
- Being denied due process
- Discrimination at sentencing, detention and release

AAIDD and ARC (2014)

Slide 15

Common Characteristics

People who have IDD and commit crimes often share common characteristics:

- have mild IDD
- have no or minimal supports
- come from lower economic status backgrounds
- are isolated from their family and community
- are often homeless

Hayes (2012)

Slide 16

Common Characteristics (cont'd)

- lack productive activity during the day
- have substance abuse problems that affect their financial situation
- have high recidivism
- have high risk of mental illness

Hayes (2012)

Slide 17

Competence to Stand Trial

Competence or fitness to stand trial refers to the ability of the person accused to participate in their own defense. It is the most common forensic assessment in the United States.

It can also be referred to as "adjudicative competency."

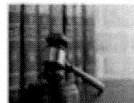

Hoge (2016)

Slide 18

Restoration of Competency

In Canada, having competency decisions appealed is done through a Review Board. Reviews of the incompetency decision must be made at regular and stipulated intervals after the initial order of incompetency to stand trial.

In the United States, a ruling of incompetency may be reversed and competency may be restored through educational interventions. Procedures in the United States vary by state.

Danzer, et al. (2020)

Slide 19

Forensic Psychiatry

Forensic psychiatry relates to the assessment, treatment and rehabilitation of people with serious mental illness who have come into contact with the law as a result of committing a crime.

After an order of unfit to stand trial has been made, the person is typically ordered to a hospital with forensic mental health treatment for mental health care.

Arboleda-Florez (2006)

Slide 20

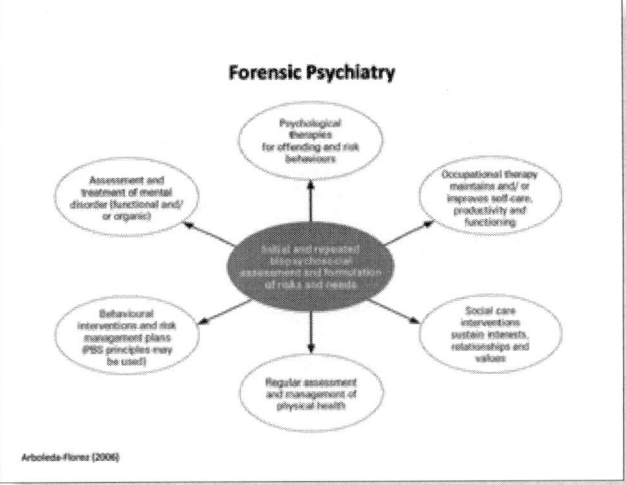

Slide 21

Court Diversion

Formal court diversion programs have been developed both in Canada and the U.S. but are not standard and generally partner with mental health courts or therapeutic courts.

How diversion is managed will typically depend specific court and availability of community services in a given area.

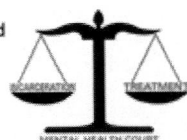

Bright (1989)

Slide 22

Court Diversion

A diversion program in the criminal justice system is a form of sentence in which the criminal offender joins a rehabilitation program, which will help remedy the behavior leading to the original arrest, allow the offender to avoid conviction and, in some jurisdictions, hide a criminal record.

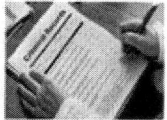

Slide 23

Court Diversion

A diversion program in the criminal justice system is a form of sentence in which the criminal offender joins a rehabilitation program, which will help remedy the behavior leading to the original arrest, allow the offender to avoid conviction and, in some jurisdictions, hide a criminal record.

In the United States, the availability of diversion programs depends upon the jurisdiction, the nature of the crime (usually nonviolent offences) and in many cases the exercise of prosecutorial discretion. The programs are often run by a police department, court, a district attorney's office or outside agency.

Slide 24

Custody/Incarceration

Offenders who have IDD might find it difficult to follow rules for a variety of reasons.

* They may not have the ability to understand the implied social rules or recall and follow more concrete rules more often than others.
* Misconduct offenses must be documented, and frequent offenses can create an accumulation of misconduct reports.

Rickford & Kimmett (2005)

Slide 25

Custody/Incarceration

Without specific training in identifying IDD and dual diagnosis in offenders, corrections officers have little opportunity to understand patterns they may observe in behavior or recommend effective plans for treatment.

Offenders with IDD are at increased risk of harm when incarcerated due to vulnerabilities to exploitation, abuse, manipulation, misunderstanding expectations and inability to benefit from most existing treatment programs in correctional facilities.

United Nations (2009)

Slide 26

Custody/Incarceration

The average length of stay in custody is frequently less than 35 days. This time period is often too short to provide effective treatment programming, particularly if the offender requires longer-than-average time to complete the program.

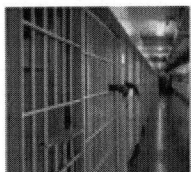

Endicott (1991)

Slide 27

Community residential settings more commonly call emergency services in response to behavioral crises. Organizationally, service providers should consider the following before developing crisis plans that include calling police:

- Is law enforcement intended to assure safety?
- Should a person with disabilities be charged with a crime for aggression to care providers?
- Or aggression toward peers?
- Is it the responsibility of the provider to manage aggressive behavior?

Slide 28

Service providers, care providers and families typically involve police services for the following reasons:

- Elopement, or the person with IDD is missing
- Generally unsafe behavior
- Failure to follow rules providers have in place
- Sexual misconduct

Slide 29

Special Needs Offenders:
Role of Special Needs Units

- Identification of vulnerable populations

- Provision of treatment while incarcerated

- Maintaining safety while incarcerated

Bright (1989)

Slide 30

Challenges within the Justice System

"Prisons are designed to provide secure containment of prisoners and to maintain order with a hope that punitive procedures will produce an inhibiting effect on criminal behavior."

However, as Gardner, et al., point out, the assumption of the system is that the offender has alternate prosocial behavior that they can choose. For people with IDD, this is often a false assumption.

Gardner, et al. (1998)

M O D U L E   1 3

Slide 31

Treatment and Rehabilitation

- Treat co-occurring disorders

- Problem-solve common issues and stressors

- Identify what role the disability has and tailor treatment accordingly

Bright (1989)

Slide 32

Treatment and Rehabilitation:
Preventing Recidivism

- Support with understanding social skills and problem-solving
- Education about following laws
- Work with impulse control, emotional regulation and problem-solving skills

D'Zurilla and Nezu (2001)

Slide 33

Assisting the Justice System
to Support Special Needs Offenders

If a person working in a corrections environment suspects a person has IDD, there are a number of interaction tips that can help build a positive rapport and increase the effectiveness of the interaction, treatment process or the person's ability to follow the rules.

Spence & Hughes (2003)

Slide 34

**Assisting the Justice System
to Support Special Needs Offenders**

- When possible, limit distractions when communicating and interacting.
- Take extra time to explain expectations.
- Do not use slang or jargon.
- Be direct and straightforward.
- Speak clearly and use precise language.

Spence & Hughes (2003)

Slide 35

**Assisting the Justice System
to Support Special Needs Offenders**

- When giving directions or orders, try not to give more than one or two steps at a time.
- Allow the person some time to process information and act on it.
- Ask the person to use their own words to explain what they think you are saying or asking.

Spence & Hughes (2003)

Slide 36

**Assisting the Justice System
to Support Special Needs Offenders**

- Use open-ended questions as opposed to yes/no questions.
- Be aware of body language being consistent with verbal communication.
- Be sensitive to the impact psychotropic medication can have on a person's ability to process information. Side effects can cause fatigue, lower ability to concentrate and impact short-term memory, which affects interviews and interactions.

Spence & Hughes (2003)

M
O
D
U
L
E

1
3

Slide 37

**Assisting the Justice System
to Support Special Needs Offenders**

- Many people with IDD are strongly motivated to do what they believe is expected of them.
- They learn to listen for certain words or inflections. They may even copy moods as they try to give "correct" answers.
- They want to be accepted by and to please others. Many have adapted by use of denial. They may affirm the last choice, agree or repeat the last word. For example:
  - Q: "Do you understand what I have told you?" A: "Told you."
  - Q: "Do you want to take a break or keep going?" A. "Keep going."

Spence & Hughes (2003)

Slide 38

Ultimately, our goals for supporting people with IDD/dual diagnosis when they come into contact with the justice system is to help them achieve the best possible outcome through treatment, rehabilitation and reintegration.

It's important to remember that the social services system is not at cross-purposes with the justice system. Each must take the opportunity to understand, advocate and educate, as appropriate, to the best possible outcome for the person involved.

M
O
D
U
L
E

1
3

Post-test

Module XIII: Justice System Considerations

_____ 1. True or false: In the early part of the twentieth century, it was an accepted theory that people who have an intellectual/developmental disability were inherently criminal in their nature.

_____ 2. This is not a reason there are challenges in capturing accurate prevalence rates of people who have an intellectual/developmental disability who interact with the justice system:
(a) Underreporting to police services
(b) Stats tend to represent the arrest and conviction rate as opposed to the true offending prevalence
(c) People with IDD rarely get arrested
(d) Research more often focuses on the rates of recidivism as opposed to the rates of offending

_____ 3. Counterfeit criminality is:
(a) The concept that criminal behavior is performed for reasons other than criminality or criminal gain
(b) The concept that a person with IDD can appear innocent even if they are guilty of committing a crime
(c) When someone is falsely accused of a crime
(d) The same as bait-and-switch, which is unethical but not always illegal

_____ 4. Which of the following is not considered an effective means to support people who have IDD in avoiding criminal behavior?
(a) Assist people in developing friendships and learning about different types of social interactions
(b) Ensure people are aware of the laws in their state/province so they can avoid breaking the law
(c) Ensure people have an opportunity to advocate for themselves in ways they want
(d) Provide an opportunity for people to practice social skills in a variety of situations and environments

_____ 5. True or false: A person who has IDD frequently has specific vulnerabilities that can lead to initial involvement with the justice system and faces challenges that can often make it difficult to end that involvement or avoid future involvement.

M
O
D
U
L
E

1
3

_____ 6. When people who have an IDD become involved with the justice system, they frequently experience prejudice, lack of understanding and fear. They often experience difficulties with:

(a) Not being recognized as having a disability

(b) Being victimized at high rates

(c) Being denied opportunities for reparation

(d) All of the above

(e) (a) and (c) only

_____ 7. Fill in the blank: Fitness to stand trial, or _____ , refers to the ability of a person accused to participate in their own defense.

_____ 8. Forensic psychiatry relates to:

(a) Understanding the behavior and motivation of people who commit homicide

(b) Assessment and treatment of dangerous psychopaths

(c) The assessment, treatment and rehabilitation of people with serious mental illness who have come in contact with the law as a result of committing a crime

(d) The gathering and analysis of all crime-related psychological and psychiatric evidence in order to come to a conclusion about a suspect

_____ 9. True or false: A diagnosis of IDD and a mental illness means a person will be found unfit to stand trial.

_____ 10. Which of the following is not an ethical consideration that should be discussed before caregivers and service providers develop crisis plans that include calling police services:

(a) Is it the responsibility of the provider to manage aggressive behavior?

(b) Should a person who has IDD be charged for aggression to caregivers or providers?

(c) What is the goal of the intervention?

(d) What is the caregiver's or service provider's expectation of police services?

(e) None of the above

MODULE 13

Supplemental Materials

Module XIII: Justice System Considerations

Think about the traits or characteristics of the people you support. Are they vulnerable to involvement with the justice system?

What factors lead you to conclude the person is vulnerable?

1. _____

2. _____

3. _____

4. _____

5. _____

6. _____

How can you support the person, or what strategies would you develop to address these vulnerabilities?

_____

_____

Does your community have a formal relationship with justice services in your area? Is there a network or committee that works on building mutual understanding and bridges across sectors?

_____

_____

Can you develop a collaborative relationship with justice professionals in your area? How would you build that relationship? What goals would you have for this endeavor?

_____

Strategies for Interacting with a Special Needs Offender

If you are interacting with someone you know has an IDD, or if you have reason to suspect the person may have an IDD, here are some suggestions to assist with building rapport and increasing the effectiveness of the interaction with the person.

- Find a place to communicate that is free of as many distractions as possible.

- Confirm you have the person's attention and take extra time to explain expectations.

- Be direct and use straightforward language when communicating. Avoid the use of acronyms, jargon and slang.

- Speak clearly and be aware of the rate and rhythm of your speech (cadence). Use clear, precise language. Many people who have IDD can find abstract concepts and communication challenging to interpret. Abstract ideas, metaphors and common expressions of speech can be quite challenging to interpret.

- Be specific when giving directions. Explain clearly and demonstrate, if possible, what you want them to do. You may need to explain how to complete the request you make. If the person is able to read, try writing down instructions, as they may have more difficulty retaining information that is shared verbally or following verbal directions.

- Also, when giving directions that involve two or more steps or components, offer one or two steps at a time. A person who has an IDD may have difficulty processing several steps in a process at a time. If this is the case, they may have difficulty remembering all the steps or become overwhelmed and not complete all the directions given.

- Use visual cues that help the person understand what you are saying. Visual cues help a person understand the words they are hearing.

- Allow a person time to process information and act on it. A person who has an IDD may need additional time to understand what is being said before responding or taking action.

- Check the person's understanding of the information they receive or any instructions given. It is not uncommon for people with an IDD to echo the words they have heard or indicate agreement/assent when they do not understand or agree with information. By asking the person to use their own words to explain what you have said, you will get a clear picture of what the person understands.

- Use open-ended questions to avoid yes and no answers. Some people who have an IDD will answer the way they think you want them to answer.

- Be aware of your body language. Make sure your verbal messages and your body language are consistent. For example, if you are saying that you are not upset but your arms are crossed over your chest and your facial expression is grimacing, you may physically appear angry. It can be difficult for a person who has an IDD to interpret the contrasting messages.

Reference: Spence, D. & Hughes, J. (2003). An Instructor Manual for Training Staff Who Work with People Who Have Mental Health Needs and A Developmental Disability. Behaviour Management Services York and Simcoe

Fetal Alcohol Spectrum Disorder (FASD)

According to an article in the International Journal of Law and Psychiatry, "One of the common adverse outcomes associated with FASD is criminal justice system (CJS) involvement, and individuals with FASD are believed to be over-represented in forensic and correctional settings. The FASD population is an exceptionally heterogeneous and complex group, with varying life experiences, clinical profiles, and levels of functional ability. These factors likely impact how an individual with FASD might engage with the CJS, function within the system, and respond to justice-related supports and intervention initiatives."

Reference: Flannigan, K., Pei, J., Stewart M., & Johnson, Fetal Alcohol Spectrum Disorder and the Criminal Justice System: A systematic literature review. Int J Law Psychiatry, 57, 42-52, Elsevier, 2018.

There are some patterns in offenses and behaviors that can indicate a person may have FASD.

- Repetitive but non-escalating pattern of repeat offenses over short- and long-term periods.

- Offenses exacerbated by drugs and/or alcohol.

- Warnings, probation, prison time do not act as deterrents for future offenses.

- Often numerous charges for the same offense.

- The person may appear to have no remorse.

- The person will "talk the talk" but may be unable to "walk the walk" without support.

M
O
D
U
L
E

1
3

Justice professionals may experience the following challenges when working with a person who has FASD:

- An unreliable memory may result in changes to the person's "story."

- The person will agree to leading questions/sentences.

- Planning capacity and impulse control are often impaired, which means the person is more likely to commit offenses of opportunity and impulse such as shoplifting, break and enter, car theft, etc.

- FASD causes impairment in executive function so the person may have difficulty predicting the outcome or consequences of their actions or problem-solve solutions.

Reference: Streissguth AP, Barr HM, Kogan J, Bookstein FL. Understanding the occurrence of secondary disabilities in clients with fetal alcohol syndrome (FAS) and Fetal Alcohol Effects (FAE): Final report. 1996; Seattle: University of Washington Publication Services.

Autism Spectrum Disorders

Tips for Positive Interactions

1. Allow time for the person to acclimatize to the new environment. If it is safe to do so, allow the person to wander and touch objects if they need to do so.

2. Do not expect eye contact or force it from the person.

3. Do not interfere with self-rocking, hand-flapping, twirling, etc. These behaviors can help people calm themselves.

4. Model behavior you want to see from the person.

5. Personal space is subjective. Be prepared for the person to invade the personal space of others as their own may be different.

6. Keep communication brief, clear and literal. Try to frame demand/requests in terms of what the person needs to do as opposed to what they need to stop doing, e.g., give the direction "stand by the door" instead of "stop pacing around the room."

7. Give the person extra time to answer or comply after a command or question.

8. Tell the person the rules: the formal and informal rules. People who have an ASD often learn to rely on and respect rules. Routine and rules can be natural strengths for people who have an ASD when they understand what the routines and rules are.

9. Avoid sarcasm, joking or teasing.

10. Try to reduce outside stimulation when possible.

Reference: Children's Hospital and Health System (2009). Autism Spectrum Disorders: A Special Needs Response Guide for Police Officers. Milwaukee, Wisconsin.

Recommended Resources

Offenders with Dual Diagnosis: Intellectual Developmental Disabilities/Autism Spectrum Disorders & Psychiatric Disorder, https://www.porticonetwork.ca/documents/623998/2052895/ CAMH+FDDSS+Offenders+with+IDD-ASD+Sept+2019.pdf/3317c858-0499-495b-a9f6-b0acc64320f7.

Lindsay, et al., *The Wiley Handbook on What Works for Offenders with Intellectual and Developmental Disabilities: An Evidence-Based Approach to Theory, Assessment, and Treatment* (New York: Wiley, 2019).

Søndenaa, E., Olsen, T., Kermit, P.S., Dahl, N.C. and Envik, R. (2019), "Intellectual disabilities and offending behaviour: the awareness and concerns of the police, district attorneys and judges," *Journal of Intellectual Disabilities and Offending Behaviour*, Vol. 10 No. 2, pp. 34-42. https://doi.org/10.1108/ JIDOB-04-2019-0007.

J. Paul Fedoroff, Deborah Richards, Rebekah Ranger, Susan Curry, The predictive validity of common risk assessment tools in men with intellectual disabilities and problematic sexual behaviors, *Research in Developmental Disabilities*, Volume 57, 2016, Pages 29-38, ISSN 0891-4222, https://doi.org/10.1016/j. ridd.2016.06.011.

The Arc—Criminal Justice Initiatives, https://thearc.org/our-initiatives/criminal-justice/

M
O
D
U
L
E

1
3

Module XIV

The Importance
of Direct Support Professionals

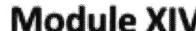

Pre-test

Module XIV: The Importance of Direct Support Professionals

_____ 1. In general, _____ spend more time with the person with IDD/MI than any other team member and can make a big difference in the quality of life for people.
(a) Behavior specialists
(b) Psychiatrists
(c) Direct support professionals
(d) Pharmacists

_____ 2. Luke wants to try out for the community theater since he was in his high school play and he misses performing. His mom doesn't want him to go to auditions because Luke has depression and she is concerned that rejection will trigger a mental health crisis. How can Luke's Direct Support Professional best support Luke?
(a) Talk with Luke about different options and prepare him for possible outcomes
(b) Call to schedule a psychiatrist's appointment in anticipation of increased need for medication
(c) Partner with Luke's mom to find a more realistic goal for him
(d) Offer Luke a preferred activity if he skips the audition

_____ 3. True or false: When we include Direct Support Professionals in planning for persons with IDD/MI, more accurate and useful information will emerge.

_____ 4. Identify a workforce challenge(s) in the field of IDD/MI:
(a) Most Direct Support Professionals are not certified or credentialed
(b) Requirements for employment vary according to agency or employer
(c) Direct Support Professionals generally work for low wages
(d) All of the above

_____ 5. The NADSP Code of Ethics®:
(a) Is intended to serve as a straightforward and relevant guide for Direct (b) Support Professionals to help resolve the ethical dilemmas they face every day
(c) Encourages Direct Support Professionals to achieve the highest ideals of the profession
(d) Includes the principles of confidentiality, respect, self-determination and advocacy
(e) All of the above

_____ 6. Which of the following is not a challenge many Direct Support Professionals face in their work?
(a) A lot is expected from Direct Support Professionals who are often left out of the planning process
(b) Direct Support Professionals are unwilling to participate in training
(c) Direct Support Professionals are often required to implement, maintain, evaluate and assess plans they did not develop
(d) Some Direct Support Professionals are expected to use tools with which they are not familiar

_____ 7. _____ helps staff learn and practice skills in the setting where they will be used.
(a) Classroom training
(b) Virtual courses
(c) On-the-job training
(d) Certification

_____ 8. The goal of programs such as the NADD Direct Support Professional Certification and the Ontario Developmental Services Human Resource Strategy is to build capacity among workforce professionals through a set of standards called:
(a) Core competencies
(b) Requirements
(c) Expectations
(d) Learning skills

_____ 9. True or false: Training is not complete until a Direct Support Professional can demonstrate the skill on the job.

_____ 10. An outcome(s) of Direct Support Professionals who demonstrate competency in IDD/MI include:
(a) Greater consistency and efficacy in support delivery for people with mental and behavioral health needs
(b) More turnover and lower wages for Direct Support Professionals who work in the field of IDD/MI
(c) Direct Support Professionals are less empowered to provide feedback and contribute to planning
(d) Direct Support Professionals who require more supervision

MODULE 14

Slide 1

Module XIV

**The Importance
of Direct Support Professionals**

Slide 2

Learning Objectives

- Recognize the role of Direct Support Professionals (DSPs) in providing quality supports to people with IDD/MI.
- Identify several workforce challenges of Direct Support Professionals.
- Recognize importance in building competency to ensure quality supports.

Slide 3

1. The role of the DSP
2. Workforce challenges
3. Including and empowering DSPs
4. Building competency
5. Supporting a competent workforce

Slide 4

Direct Support Professionals (DSPs) spend more time with the person with IDD/MI than any other professional. The competence of the DSP can make a big difference in the quality of life for people.

Slide 5

The Role of the DSP in IDD/MI

- DSPs are often the ones charged with supporting skill building.
- They help the person engage in recommended therapies on a day-to-day basis.
- Using the word "professional" acknowledges the respected role of these persons in the community at large and makes the point that DSPs are valued caretakers.

Slide 6

Including DSPs in Planning

DSPs work closest with individuals and often determine the success and efficacy of interventions related to:

- Behavior planning
- Health and wellness
- Skill acquisition
- Employment and recreation
- Relationship building

M
O
D
U
L
E

1
4

Slide 7

Exercise

Consider the many ways DSPs have an impact in their roles at your program/agency.

How is this different for people with IDD/MI?

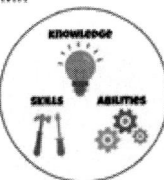

Slide 8

Workforce Challenges

- DSPs generally are not certified or credentialed.
- Requirements for employment vary.
- DSPs have varying levels of education.
- Educational opportunities are often limited.
- DSPs generally work for low wages.
- DSPs' work experience is diverse.

Slide 9

Training Challenges

- A lot is expected from staff who are often left out of the planning process.
- Required to implement, maintain, evaluate and assess plans they did not develop.
- Do not understand the cause of behavior or the goal of the plan, only given "strategy."
- Expected to use tools they are not familiar with.
- Passive role (instructed by "experts").

Slide 10

Supervision Challenges

- Lack of support from managers.
- Limited resources.
- Staff turnover causes diversion from plan ("anyone can do it").
- Given directives without explanation.
- Not empowered to contribute.

Slide 11

Value of Including DSPs

- Staff often have most updated information.
- Opportunity for staff to take ownership in planning for the individuals they support.
- More likely to follow plans and strategies if involved in development.
- Increases staff efficacy in following plans or implementing strategies.

Slide 12

Value of Including DSPs

- Greater consistency in support delivery.
- Staff learn to be more observant and more comfortable contributing information.
- More accurate and useful information will emerge.
- Individuals will associate staff with progress, and challenging behavior will decrease.

M
O
D
U
L
E

1
4

Slide 13

How Do We Empower Staff to Participate?

Activity: Using the ideas below, brainstorm ways to include DSPs in support planning.

- Ask DSPs for feedback, then listen.
- Change approach, welcome cooperation.
- Establish trusting relationships.
- Provide technical assistance and demonstrations.
- Show progress and include staff in modifications.
- Address requests in a timely manner.
- Be conscious of staff cultural diversity and concerns.

Slide 14

DSPs: Building Capacity

- Classroom and online trainings
- Team meetings
- On-the-job practice
- Mentoring and modeling
- Evidence-based skill standards
- DSP core competencies
- Credentialing programs

Slide 15

NADD Direct Support Professional Certification

NADD has developed the NADD Competency-Based Direct Support Professional Certification Program to certify the competency of DSPs who support people with a dual diagnosis.

- Acknowledge the importance of the DSP in providing treatment and support to people with IDD/MI.
- Increase the capacity of DSPs to work with individuals with IDD/MI.

Slide 16

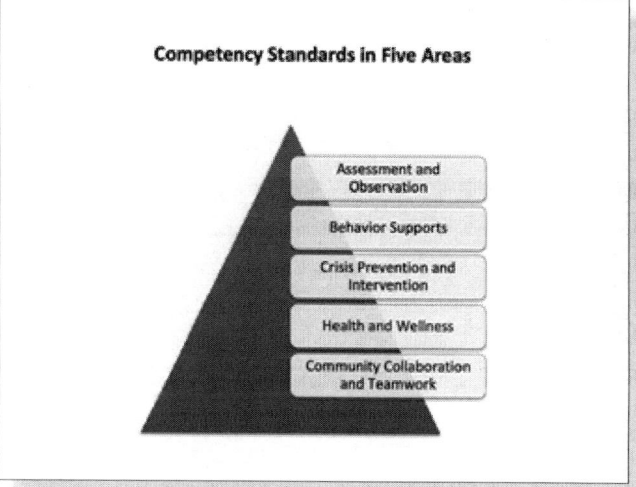

Competency Standards in Five Areas

Assessment and Observation

Behavior Supports

Crisis Prevention and Intervention

Health and Wellness

Community Collaboration and Teamwork

Slide 17

Core Competency

The Developmental Services Human Resources Strategy identified the core competencies of Direct Support Professionals, Direct Support Supervisors, Specialized Support Workers, Clinical Specialists, Managers and Directors.

The DSHR Strategy work also identified definitions and a process by which each competency can be measured and encouraged within each position.

Provincial Network on Developmental Services , Ontario, 2020

Slide 18

Core Competency

In Ontario, the Developmental Services Human Resource Strategy has taken a multipronged approach to achieving its goals to:

- Increase pool of qualified developmental services professionals.
- Ensure consistency in education, training and professional development in Ontario's developmental services sector.
- Provide opportunity for a variety of career paths for developmental service professionals.
- Enhance management expertise.

Provincial Network on Developmental Services , Ontario, 2020

Slide 19

Core Competency

Through collaborative work between the Ministry of Community and Social Services and the Provincial Network on Developmental Services, 15 core competencies and four threshold competencies were identified.

The work on core competencies included identifying a training and performance management process for Direct Support Professionals, Managers, Directors and Executive Directors within developmental services organizations. It further developed training for Human Resources professionals on how to embed competencies into HR practices.

Provincial Network on Developmental Services , Ontario, 2020

Slide 20

Core Competencies

Advocating for Others	Collaboration
Creative Problem-Solving and Decision-Making	Developing Others
Fostering Independence in Others	Holding People Accountable
Initiative	Interpersonal Relationships and Respect
Leading Others	Managing Change
Relationship and Network Building	Resilience
Resource Management	Self-Development
Strategic Thinking	

The Hay Group, 2009

Slide 21

Threshold Competencies

Flexibility	Self-Control
Service Orientation	Values and Ethics

The Hay Group, 2009

MODULE 14

Slide 22

NADSP Code of Ethics

- Person-Centered Supports
- Promoting Physical and Emotional Well-Being
- Integrity and Responsibility
- Confidentiality
- Justice, Fairness, Equity
- Respect
- Relationships
- Self-Determination
- Advocacy

Slide 23

Activity: David's dream is to go on a vacation to California to visit his brother. He is afraid to fly and barely has enough money to pay his current bills. After learning about this dream, his DSP should:

A. Focus on helping David recognize that he cannot possibly save enough for the trip.

B. Call David's brother and ask him to visit David's home instead. It's more practical and cost-effective.

C. Help David plan a more affordable vacation at a nearby resort.

D. Encourage David to develop a plan to reach his dream by assisting him with budgeting money and addressing his flying anxiety through desensitization.

Slide 24

Beyond Training

- Training is not complete until staff can demonstrate the skill on the job.
- Develop methods and documents to evaluate and demonstrate competency.
- Consider how to apply the NADSP Code of Ethics® when faced with competing demands and expectations.

M
O
D
U
L
E

1
4

Slide 25

Effective Team Process

- Design team meetings to prioritize and solve problems; use competency areas as the roadmap to generate solutions.
- Identify how to modify plans in response to the changing behavioral and psychiatric needs of the persons served.
- Prepare individuals and information for appointments with health professionals.
- Set expectation of DSP contribution and feedback.

Slide 26

Recognizing Excellence

- Recognize DSPs who deliver quality care to individuals with IDD/MI.
- Promote best practice in IDD/MI across agencies and settings.
- Encourage other DSPs to aspire to competency.
- Develop career pathway for DSPs.
- Provide support from supervisors and peers.
- Promote current DSPs to leadership roles to learn the needs of the persons supported.

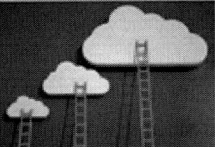

Slide 27

Building Competency: Outcomes

- DSPs feel valued and take pride in the direct support work provided to individuals who have IDD/MI.
- DSPs are recognized for the skills, knowledge and values they have acquired in the field of dual diagnosis.
- By utilizing competency standards as guidelines, staff are empowered and valued.
- Greater consistency and efficacy in support delivery for people with mental and behavioral health needs.

Post-test

Module XIV: The Importance of Direct Support Professionals

_____ 1. In general, _____ spend more time with the person with IDD/MI than any other team member and can make a big difference in the quality of life for people.
(a) Behavior specialists
(b) Psychiatrists
(c) Direct support professionals
(d) Pharmacists

_____ 2. Luke wants to try out for the community theater since he was in his high school play and he misses performing. His mom doesn't want him to go to auditions because Luke has depression and she is concerned that rejection will trigger a mental health crisis. How can Luke's Direct Support Professional best support Luke?
(a) Talk with Luke about different options and prepare him for possible outcomes
(b) Call to schedule a psychiatrist's appointment in anticipation of increased need for medication
(c) Partner with Luke's mom to find a more realistic goal for him
(d) Offer Luke a preferred activity if he skips the audition

_____ 3. True or false: When we include Direct Support Professionals in planning for persons with IDD/MI, more accurate and useful information will emerge.

_____ 4. Identify a workforce challenge(s) in the field of IDD/MI:
(a) Most Direct Support Professionals are not certified or credentialed
(b) Requirements for employment vary according to agency or employer
(c) Direct Support Professionals generally work for low wages
(d) All of the above

_____ 5. The NADSP Code of Ethics®:
(a) Is intended to serve as a straightforward and relevant guide for Direct (b) Support Professionals to help resolve the ethical dilemmas they face every day
(c) Encourages Direct Support Professionals to achieve the highest ideals of the profession
(d) Includes the principles of confidentiality, respect, self-determination and advocacy
(e) All of the above

MODULE 14

_____ 6. Which of the following is not a challenge many Direct Support Professionals face in their work?

(a) A lot is expected from Direct Support Professionals who are often left out of the planning process

(b) Direct Support Professionals are unwilling to participate in training

(c) Direct Support Professionals are often required to implement, maintain, evaluate and assess plans they did not develop

(d) Some Direct Support Professionals are expected to use tools with which they are not familiar

_____ 7. _____ helps staff learn and practice skills in the setting where they will be used.

(a) Classroom training

(b) Virtual courses

(c) On-the-job training

(d) Certification

_____ 8. The goal of programs such as the NADD Direct Support Professional Certification and the Ontario Developmental Services Human Resource Strategy is to build capacity among workforce professionals through a set of standards called:

(a) Core competencies

(b) Requirements

(c) Expectations

(d) Learning skills

_____ 9. True or false: Training is not complete until a Direct Support Professional can demonstrate the skill on the job.

_____ 10. An outcome(s) of Direct Support Professionals who demonstrate competency in IDD/MI include:

(a) Greater consistency and efficacy in support delivery for people with mental and behavioral health needs

(b) More turnover and lower wages for Direct Support Professionals who work in the field of IDD/MI

(c) Direct Support Professionals are less empowered to provide feedback and contribute to planning

(d) Direct Support Professionals who require more supervision

Supplemental Materials

Module XIV: The Importance of Direct Support Professionals

Consider the many ways Direct Support Professionals (DSPs) have an impact on the lives of people with IDD/MI. What knowledge, skills and abilities are essential to supporting people with behavior and mental health needs?

Direct Support Professionals are valuable members of behavior and mental health support teams. List some strategies to encourage DSPs to feel empowered to contribute and participate.

Consider these guidelines below.

- Be mindful of staff cultural diversity and concerns.

- Consider preferred communication methods.

- Use team meetings to prioritize staff concerns.

- Create a partnership with individuals with IDD/MH needs.

- Address requests in a timely manner.

Discussion: What are barriers to receiving participation from DSPs? How can we address these obstacles?

Activity: Reflect on your own work. How can you improve your knowledge of other service systems to facilitate effective collaboration within your agency or across agency boundaries to improve outcomes for someone you support with IDD/MI?
What do you need to do this?
Who is a potential partner or resource?

MODULE 14

Below are some things DSPs can help monitor to support collaboration with other health professionals. Treatment coordination and information gathering:

- Appetite

- Sleep pattern

- Changes in mood

- Observed side effects

- Clarification of dosing

- Changes in behavior & symptoms

- Symptoms

Instructions and expectations from a prescriber to share and support person with IDD/MI:

- How long will it take? What changes to look for and when?

- What positive changes should be expected?

- Possible side effects

- Diet restrictions or other considerations (e.g., alcohol, grapefruit)

Resource: *Accompanying an Individual to the Doctor: Tips for Direct Support Professionals and other Caregivers*: https://iddtoolkit.vkcsites.org/wp-content/uploads/accompanytodr18.pdf

Here is a list of ways to support people during health appointments and with medication management.

- Be a partner and advocate during appointments.

- Encourage and support the person to be informed and prepared to speak at the appointment.

- Support data-driven recommendations (document change in symptoms).

- Communicate the patient and team's ideas, concerns and expectations.

MODULE 14

- Monitor the outcomes of treatment, both beneficial and adverse.

- Assist people to know their medications to the best of their ability.

- Document prescribing decisions, the reasons for medication and expected outcomes.

- Always explain medication changes and why and monitoring is important.

- Educate the importance of avoiding alcohol, certain foods, and risks (suddenly discontinuing medications, etc.).

Activity: Direct Support Professionals often receive a great deal of training as part of their job responsibilities. What are some ways we can make sure DSPs are using what they learn to better support people with IDD/MI?

Recommended Resources

National Alliance for Direct Support. (2016). *Direct Support Professional Competency Areas: The Foundation of Direct Support Practice.* Albany, NY: NADSP: https://www.nadsp.org/15-competency-areas/

National Alliance for Direct Support Code of Ethics: https://www.nadsp.org/wp-content/uploads/2017/04/Code-of-Ethics-fillable-form-2016.pdf

NADD Competency-Based IDD/MI Dual Diagnosis Direct Support Professional Certification Program Competency Areas: https://thenadd.org/dsp-certification-competency-areas/

Developmental Services Human Resource Strategy Core Competencies: http://www.ontariodevelopmentalservices.ca/resources/core-competencies

National Frontline Supervisor Competencies - Research & Training Center on Community Living Institute on Community Integration (UCEDD): https://rtc.umn.edu/docs/National_Frontline_Supervisor_comp_7-2-13.pdf

MHDD National Training Center courses: https://www.mhddcenter.org/learn-now/

M
O
D
U
L
E

1
4

Worksheets and Forms to complete along with people with ID/MH: https://thenadd.org/materials-for-positive-identity-development/

Invaluable: The Unrecognized Profession of Direct Support: https://ici.umn.edu/product/invaluable/resources

M
O
D
U
L
E

1
4

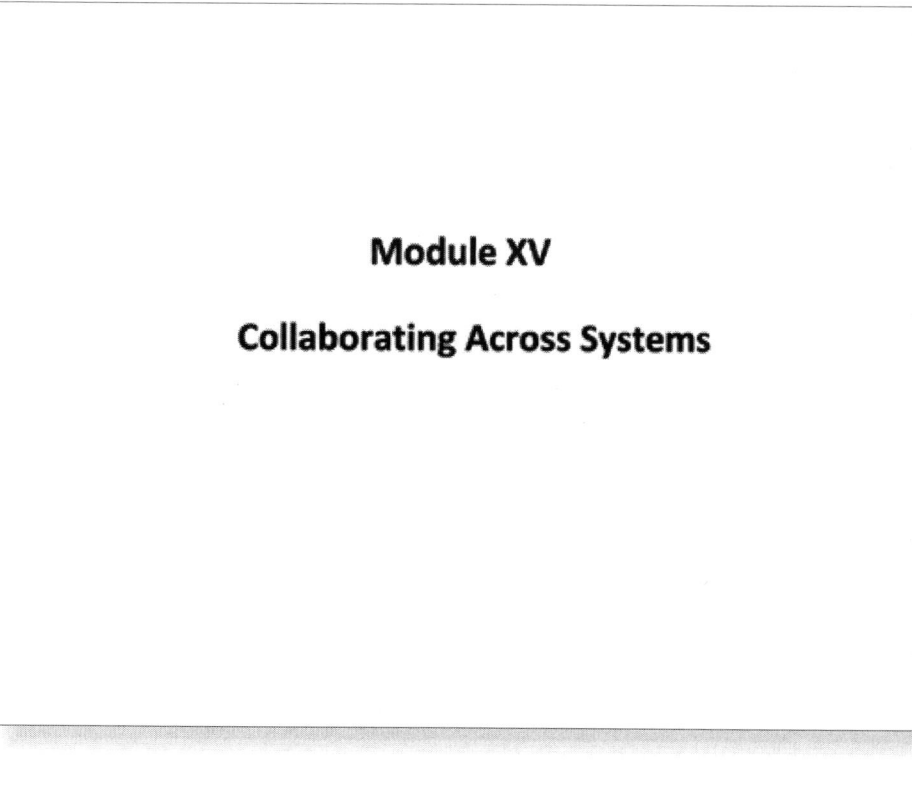

Module XV

Collaborating Across Systems

Pre-test

Module XV: Collaborating Across Systems

_____ 1. Lack of strategic planning has led to a "silo system" that:
(a) Provides a plan to use state agencies as support
(b) Confines people with a dual diagnosis to small areas
(c) Ensures that people can escape the hustle and bustle of the city
(d) Results in access barriers to required services

_____ 2. The MH and IDD systems:
(a) Often do not collaborate, fostering divide between them
(b) May work together if the person pursues
(c) Will collaborate if the person requires treatment
(d) Always actively collaborate for betterment

_____ 3. Services for people with a dual diagnosis need to be:
(a) Based primarily on a comprehensive assessment
(b) Based primarily on the mental health concerns
(c) Based primarily on what services are available
(d) Based primarily on the level of ID

_____ 4. True or false: Dual diagnosis planning principles are based only on MH or IDD diagnoses.

_____ 5. A holistic approach to care and treatment requires:
(a) Neither a mental health nor a developmental disabilities approach
(b) A focus on a mental health approach
(c) A focus primarily on developmental disabilities
(d) Both a focus on mental health and developmental disabilities

_____ 6. Intersystem collaboration means:
(a) Interacting with your agency colleagues
(b) Interacting with the person being served
(c) Interacting with staff from other systems
(d) Interacting with the individual and their family

_____ 7. The goal of community collaboration is to:
    (a) Improve access to and availability of human services
    (b) Raise awareness for individuals within a community
    (c) Build a more effective system for individuals
    (d) All of the above

_____ 8. Co-occurring disorders should be treated:
    (a) By the severity of the disorder, with the more severe being treated first
    (b) There is no such thing as co-existing disorders
    (c) As multiple primary disorders, with each requiring active treatment and supports
    (d) By the severity of the disorder, with the milder disorders being dealt with first

_____ 9. People with a dual diagnosis generally:
    (a) Experience difficulty fitting into both systems
    (b) Can never fit into either system
    (c) Easily fit into the MH system
    (d) Easily fit into the IDD system

_____ 10. The purpose of a Dual Diagnosis Committee includes:
    (a) Using the courts to catalyze change
    (b) Protecting persons with a disability abroad
    (c) Gathering relevant information to analyze strengths/weaknesses
    (d) Building an international headquarters for people with a dual diagnosis

MODULE 15

M
O
D
U
L
E

1
5

Slide 1

Module XV

Collaborating Across Systems

Slide 2

Inter-Systems Collaboration

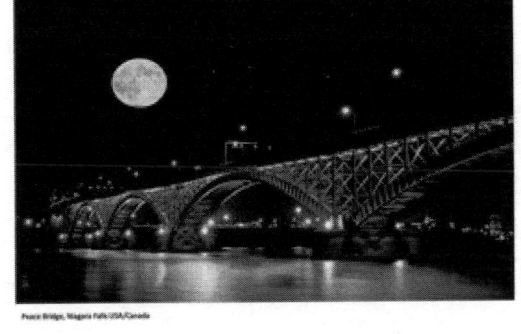

Peace Bridge, Niagara Falls USA/Canada

Slide 3

Learning Objectives

- Discuss how limited collaboration between mental health and IDD systems can result in barriers to service delivery.

- Recognize that assessment of individual need is at the center of effective person-centered service planning for individuals with MI/IDD.

- Identify the four planning and practice elements essential to working together and the factors that make each of these achievable.

Slide 4

Collaborating Across Systems

- Barriers to service delivery

- Principles in service planning

- Community collaboration and teamwork

- A framework to promote cross-system collaboration

- Service planning recommendations

Slide 5

Barriers to Service Delivery

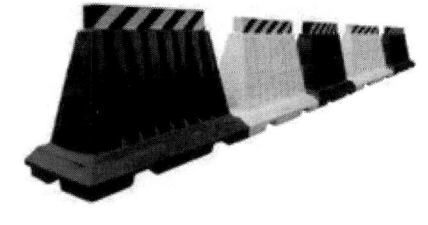

Slide 6

Dual Diagnosis Policy Barriers

The Typical Picture:

Individuals with MI and IDD are among the most challenging
persons served by both MH and IDD service delivery systems.

Moseley, 2004

Slide 7

Discussion:

Think about your experience.

How do systems barriers or gaps contribute to unmet needs of people with IDD/MI?

Slide 8

The Typical Picture:
- Failure to plan services
- Failure to fund flexible services
- Failure to obtain technical assistance

Mosely, 2004

Slide 9

The Typical Picture:

- MH providers perceive that they do not have the skills to serve adults or children with a dual diagnosis.
- IDD providers do not understand the services the MH sector offers.
- MH providers do not understand the services the IDD sector offers.

M
O
D
U
L
E

1
5

Slide 10

MH System	IDD System
• Short-term episodic treatment	• Services/supports over lifetime
• Focus on psychiatric needs	• Emphasis on direct support
• Recovery model	• Self-determination
• Local authority	• State authority
• Medication treatment	• Behavioral support (PBS)
• Consumer/client /patient	• Self-advocate/consumer

←———— **Little Collaboration** ————→

Slide 11

Institutions Provided Care in These Disciplines:

- OT
- PT
- Speech
- Psychology
- Medical
- Dental
- Other

Slide 12

From Institutionalization to Home and Community:
Complexities Challenging Community Support Systems

Complex Support Profile/Issues	Challenges
Individual with relatively minor support needs for typical daily living needs but with diagnosis of borderline personality disorder	• Frequent staffing changes throughout the day more challenging, but may be necessary • Professional oversight of interventions as often as needed • Professional help for support staff to sustain the challenges daily and consistently implement needed intervention strategies
Individuals with anticipated needs for crisis services	• Quick access to crisis services by professionals familiar with the individual and his/her needs
Individual with a dual diagnosis who needs medication, behavioral strategies and instructions for family/staff support	• Coordination of medication changes/needs with implementation of behavioral strategies • Clear guidelines on which professional to seek when problems occur • Consistency in instructions to family/staff across professionals
Individual with significant medical issue and co-occurring behavioral health need	• Coordination and prioritization of needed medical interventions when behavioral issues may impact cooperation • Coordination of needed medication changes and impact on behavioral presentation and strategies

**M
O
D
U
L
E

1
5**

Slide 13

Mental Health and Developmental Disability

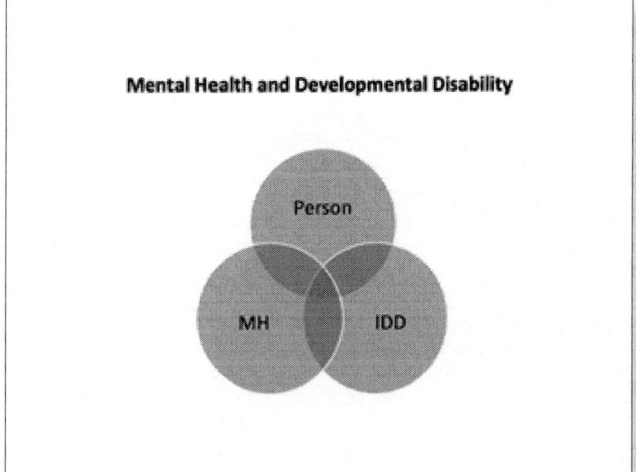

Slide 14

Cross-Systems Interface: Multiple Systems

Other systems

- Criminal justice system
- Juvenile justice system
- Educational system
- Health care system
- Substance use system
- Older adult system
- Other systems

Slide 15

Consequently, systems rarely have protocols established to plan for inter-systems collaboration. We need to advocate for inter-systems collaboration, through thoughtful inter-system planning that would support service options and funding across multiple systems.

(Kelly, 2016)

Slide 16

Principles and Practices in

Inter-Systems Service Planning

Slide 17

Dual Diagnosis Planning Principles

- Co-occurring disorders should be treated as multiple primary disorders, in which each disorder receives specific and appropriate services.
- Collaboration of appropriate services and supports must occur as needs are identified.
- Services provided to the individual are consistent with what the person wants and what supports are needed.

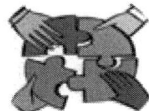

Fletcher, Beasley & Jacobson, 1999

Slide 18

Dual Diagnosis Planning Principles

- Services are determined on the basis of comprehensive assessment of the *needs* of each individual.
- Services are based on individual needs and not solely on either MH or IDD diagnosis.
- Emphasize early identification and intervention.

Fletcher, Beasley & Jacobson, 1999

Slide 19

Dual Diagnosis Planning Principles

- Involve the person and family as full partners.
- Coordinate at the system and service delivery level.

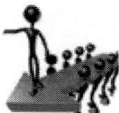

Fletcher, Beasley & Jacobson, 1999

Slide 20

Service Systems
Important Considerations

- Support access to state and local services, benefits and community-based resources.
- Recognize cultural, accessibility and linguistic barriers to service access and take steps to improve the situation.
- Advocate for a community inclusive of all citizens, including those with IDD/MI.

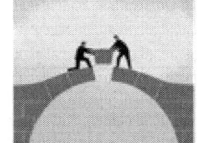

NADD-DSP

Slide 21

Facilitating Positive and Cooperative Relationships

- Navigate recommendations between systems (e.g., psychiatrists and other health professionals, employment, residential settings).
- Build positive and cooperative relationships with other health and mental health professionals.
- Work positively with multiple systems as a collaborative and cooperative member of the team.
- Maintain professional and empathetic communication and partnership with family members and friends of the individual.
- Advocate with allegiance to the individual served.

NADD, n.d.

MODULE 15

Slide 22

Discussion

During a meeting with Conner, a young adult with autism and anxiety disorder, his father is monopolizing the conversation and answering for his son.

Topics including choosing a college, auditioning for the community theater and an overnight camping trip. Dad is worried about Conner's ability to manage his diagnosis away from home or take the correct bus to the theater.

- How do we honor Connor's choice and respect the family?
- What other systems may be a resource?

Slide 23

Effective Planning and Practice Elements

1. Leadership
2. Effective staff
3. Effective treatment
4. Staff training

Adapted from Moseley, 2010

Slide 24

Effective Planning and Practice Elements

1. Leadership
   - Commitment
   - Clear lines of authority
   - Commitment to collaboration
   - Focus on the individual

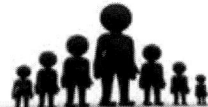

Adapted from Moseley, 2010

Slide 25

Effective Planning and Practice Elements

2. Effective Staff

- The right person
- The right match
- Build trust, dependability

- Focus on the inter-system
- Collaboration system
- IDD/MH interface

Adapted from Moseley, 2010

Slide 26

Effective Planning and Practice Elements

3. Effective Treatment
- Appropriate psychiatric diagnosis
- Effective medication treatment if needed
- Positive behavioral supports
- Effective treatment strategies such as DBT, CBT

Adapted from Moseley, 2010

Slide 27

Effective Planning and Practice Elements

4. Staff training
- DSP
- Clinicians
- Service coordinators

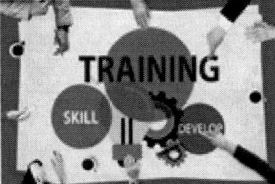

Adapted from Moseley, 2010

Slide 28

Purpose/Function of a Dual Diagnosis Committee

- Gather relevant data/information

- Identify strengths in service delivery systems

- Identify challenges/gaps in service delivery system

- Develop solutions to address challenges and gaps

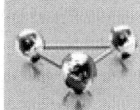

Slide 29

Stakeholders from other than MH & IDD systems could be included as appropriate. These include but are not limited to representatives from:

- Substance abuse
- Justice
- Health department
- Social services
- Parents
- Consumers
- Advocacy organizations

- Special education
- Early intervention
- Child welfare
- Coordinated children's services
- Service providers
- Senior services

Slide 30

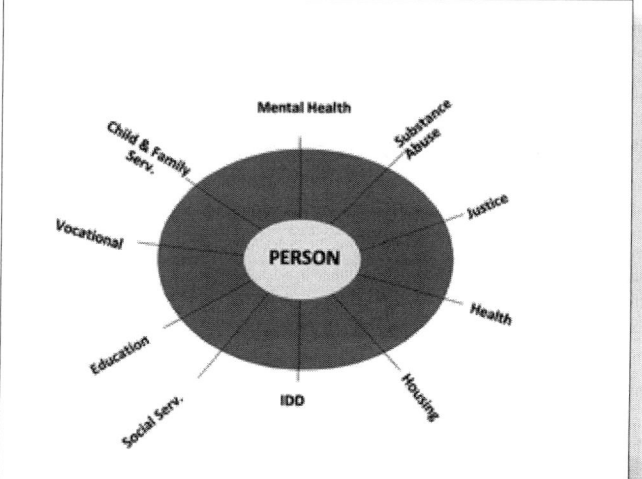

Slide 31

Improving Communication and Collaboration

Activity: Reflect on your own work and communication style. How can you improve on one of the best practices mentioned to facilitate effective collaboration within agency or across systems?

What do you need to do this?

Who is a potential ally?

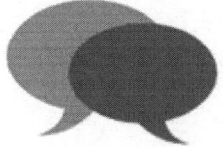

Post-test

Module XV: Collaborating Across Systems

_____ 1.   Lack of strategic planning has led to a "silo system" that:
(a) Provides a plan to use state agencies as support
(b) Confines people with a dual diagnosis to small areas
(c) Ensures that people can escape the hustle and bustle of the city
(d) Results in access barriers to required services

_____ 2.   The MH and IDD systems:
(a) Often do not collaborate, fostering divide between them
(b) May work together if the person pursues
(c) Will collaborate if the person requires treatment
(d) Always actively collaborate for betterment

_____ 3.   Services for people with a dual diagnosis need to be:
(a) Based primarily on a comprehensive assessment
(b) Based primarily on the mental health concerns
(c) Based primarily on what services are available
(d) Based primarily on the level of ID

_____ 4.   True or false: Dual diagnosis planning principles are based only on MH or IDD diagnoses.

_____ 5.   A holistic approach to care and treatment requires:
(a) Neither a mental health nor a developmental disabilities approach
(b) A focus on a mental health approach
(c) A focus primarily on developmental disabilities
(d) Both a focus on mental health and developmental disabilities

_____ 6.   Intersystem collaboration means:
(a) Interacting with your agency colleagues
(b) Interacting with the person being served
(c) Interacting with staff from other systems
(d) Interacting with the individual and their family

_____ 7. The goal of community collaboration is to:
(a) Improve access to and availability of human services
(b) Raise awareness for individuals within a community
(c) Build a more effective system for individuals
(d) All of the above

_____ 8. Co-occurring disorders should be treated:
(a) By the severity of the disorder, with the more severe being treated first
(b) There is no such thing as co-existing disorders
(c) As multiple primary disorders, with each requiring active treatment and supports
(d) By the severity of the disorder, with the milder disorders being dealt with first

_____ 9. People with a dual diagnosis generally:
(a) Experience difficulty fitting into both systems
(b) Can never fit into either system
(c) Easily fit into the MH system
(d) Easily fit into the IDD system

_____ 10. The purpose of a Dual Diagnosis Committee includes:
(a) Using the courts to catalyze change
(b) Protecting persons with a disability abroad
(c) Gathering relevant information to analyze strengths/weaknesses
(d) Building an international headquarters for people with a dual diagnosis

Supplemental Materials

Module XV: Collaborating Across Systems

In your intersystem planning meetings, it would be useful to identify and track the status of progress. Below are two tools you may find helpful. The first tool is an IDD/MI Discussion Matrix. It is intended to facilitate the planning process. The second tool is an IDD/MI Action Plan. The purpose of this tool is to identify and track action steps.

IDD/MI Discussion Matrix

	Local Level	Regional Level	State/Province Level
What is working well now in intersystem collaboration (strengths)?			
What are the major barriers to collaboration (challenges)?			
What could be done over the next year to improve collaboration (short term)?			
What could be done over the next three years to improve collaboration (long term)?			
What people/agencies need to be at the planning table?			
What person/agency will take the coordinating lead to the planning process?			
What can be done to improve collaborative relationships across systems?			
What are the next steps?			

Exercise

With regard to the above IDD/MI Discussion Matrix, please fill in the boxes to the best of your ability.

M
O
D
U
L
E

1
5

IDD/MI Action Plan

	Identified actions (goals)	Steps toward completing action (methods)	Date of expected completion	Resources needed	Responsible person(s)/ agency(ies)
Local					
Regional					
State					

MODULE 15

Exercise

With regard to the above IDD/MI Action Plan, fill in the boxes that correspond to your role, whether it be at the local, regional or state/province level.